COUNSELING DONOR FAMILY MEMBERS

Finally! After years of working as a mental health professional specializing in the emotional aspects of infertility, I have struggled to convey to my colleagues the importance of truly understanding the experience of using a donor to create a family. With one out of every eight heterosexual couples experiencing infertility and many single women and LGBT couples using a donor to conceive, it is imperative that mental health providers understand all aspects of the decision. This guide will provide insight into the world of donor-conceived families: the parent(s), children, siblings, and the donor. Our culture has promoted secrecy behind this decision and after you read this guide, you will learn how important it is for ALL parties to not live under the shroud but rather to be fully informed on how to be open and honest with no guilt or shame about the decision to donate, or to have a child or to be a donor-conceived person. Truly a must-read!!

Harriette Rovner Ferguson, LCSW, Co-author Experiencing Infertility, member of the American Society of Reproductive Medicine's Mental Health Professional Group, mental health consultant to fertility clinics

Wendy Kramer writes from the wise and compassionate perspective of a parent who has navigated the complexities of assisted reproduction. Kramer and Bertisch plant their flag firmly in support of truth and transparency for the long-term benefit of children who become adults. This book is not only a useful guide for counselors, as those considering selling their gametes to a vendor, or creating a child through assisted reproduction would be well-served to read this practical guide before making their decision.

Rich Uhrlaub, President, Adoption Search Resource Connection, Coalition for Truth and Transparency in Adoption

This is a therapist handbook that should not be put on a high shelf; it needs to be readily available. While focusing on the needs of all members of donor families, the handbook is also an intelligent, accessible, and practical guide for offering high-quality therapy to all clients who want to address issues related to their families.

Liz Margolies, LCSW and Founder, National LGBT Cancer Network

Education and competency in the issues related to donor-assisted reproduction should be required of any professional working with parents, donors, or the donor-

conceived. And by this, I mean healthcare workers, legal professionals, teachers, spiritual care workers- people who interact with humans. Especially now, as this medical technology advances its accessibility, and as more people find out later in life that they were donor-conceived. This is another intersection of diversity, equity, and inclusion for which professionals and families alike need resources for education and understanding. This handbook is just that source. As a healthcare professional, beneficiary of an egg donor, and mother to a young donor-conceived person, I can say this book is a great start. I extend gratitude to Kramer and Bertisch for their hard work in sharing this with us.

Laurie N. Baker, PhD, ABPP, Director of Psychology, Shepherd Center

Like the Donor Sibling Registry itself, this handbook is destined to be an invaluable resource. And like the DSR, it is replete with wisdom, empathy, and lived experience.

Misha Angrist, PhD, Duke University Initiative for Science & Society

This handbook relays the practical importance of this topic, particularly how mental health providers can help donor-conceived people navigate such complexities. Although discourse is shifting and stigma is decreasing, there needs to be greater awareness around assisted reproduction and its impact on individuals, couples, and families.

Dr. Elizabeth B. Lozano, Assistant Professor of Psychology and Sociology, California Northstate University

Given continued advances in assisted reproductive technologies, Counseling Donor Family Members: A Guide for Mental Health Professionals meets a critical need. Kramer and Bertisch provide a welcome and indispensable resource for practitioners, especially those working with people with infertility or seeking gamete donation, donor-conceived children, and their biological and non-biological parents. In this book, unique themes that can arise in donor family situations, such as disclosure and redefining family, are carefully and sensitively reviewed, as are the feelings and needs of all involved parties. Practical recommendations are also offered for intake assessment and talking points during therapy. This book is essential reading for therapists across a variety of settings who encounter donor family members. Students of ethics would also find this book informative and a useful reference.

Lynn A. Schaefer, Ph.D., ABPP, Fellow, American Psychological Association, Fellow, National Academy of Neuropsychology, Director of Neuropsychology, Nassau University Medical Center

This is a tangible guidebook filled with a wealth of evidence-based information as well as useful and personal anecdotes to humanize the complexities that go into donor-assisted reproduction. Not only should this be readily available to all practitioners and patients but also to all learners studying the field of reproductive medicine.

Dr. Dana Siegel, Obstetrics and Gynecology Resident, University of Colorado

I'm always struck by the parallels between the realities of donor and adoptive families, so Kramer's excellent new handbook struck very close to home. More importantly, the information and insights within it are applicable to all sorts of families. And, of course, it's necessary reading for everyone who works or might work with any member of a donor family. I think that means it's a must-read-and-use for all health professionals.

Adam Pertman, President of the National Center on Adoption and Permanency and author of *Adoption Nation*

Wendy is a true visionary and leader in this field and sheds light on subjects important for everyone involved in donor conception to understand.

Lisa Schuman, LCSW, Director, The Center for Family Building

This book is a must-read. As a mental health clinician, I find the book to be comprehensive and engaging. Each topic is well organized and coverage is in-depth. As a donor-conceived person with a rich family fabric of donor siblings, step-siblings, and adopted siblings, I found the book comforting and stabilizing. The authors share their passion and expertise in a style that is practical, accessible, and applicable.

James Holmes, LCSW

Omg, I would have begged for this in the 2000s. Thank God I had you. You were my lifeline once we found the connection, after lots of years of strife!

Parent of a Donor-Conceived Child

Wendy Kramer has long fought for openness and disclosure in the donor conception world. Having spoken to many thousands of trailblazers — and having been one herself — she offers guidance to today's counsellors on how to help people navigate this challenging terrain.
Alison Motluk, Freelance journalist and publisher of *HeyReprotech*, a weekly newsletter about assisted reproduction

Kramer and Bertisch's groundbreaking handbook details the common, but often unspoken and profound impact of assisted reproductive technologies on the lived experiences of donor-conceived children, their parents, and other family members. By weaving quantitative and qualitative data, as well as clinical insights and personal narratives, the book provides a compelling and accessible framework to help families navigate the cognitive and psychological aspects of assisted reproductive technology. Their book fills a much-needed gap for recognizing and addressing these issues that are deeply rooted in the core of the families' evolution.
Suzie Bertisch, MD, MPH

The world of donor gamete conception is novel for many mental health professionals and becoming well-informed about the unique features of donor families can be challenging as practitioners begin working with this population. This guide provides a concise overview of the unique historical, social and emotional aspects of donor gamete conception for all parties involved and advises counselors about how to navigate exceptional psychosocial realities that each member will face. This text utilizes a breadth of research, professional and personal experiences to make a compelling argument for understanding what is currently known about the challenges donor families face as they attempt to foster and maintain distal yet uniquely intimate relationships among biological and non-biological members.

Wendy Kramer has been a trailblazer in the world of donor conception for over 20 years. As the co-founder of one of the largest donor family organizations, she passionately advocates for supporting and educating families to be well-informed as they navigate donor conception. She uses her unique positionality as a biological mother of a donor-conceived child and pioneer in the field of connecting donor families to highlight the gravity of the psychological complexities for donor families.

A strength of the text is that it is well-organized and structurally appealing for any learner. The language used is easy to understand as the authors clearly define terms used and avoid medical jargon. The chapters are organized in such a way that scaffolds seminal topics such as disclosure, legal and medical concerns, problems perpetuated by gamete vendors, and the inevitable loss of anonymity with commercialized DNA technologies. Chapters 2 through 6 specifically describe the different perspectives of each member of the donor family, which makes it easy to reference a particular client type. Additionally, the bulleted format allows for information to be accessed with ease and quick reference. The inclusion of references at the end of each chapter, rather than at the end of the book, allows the reader to source relevant literature as needed. Another strength is the author's inclusion of direct quotes from donor family members. These anecdotes are captivating and heart-wrenching, as they truly evoke empathy from the reader. The quotes also offer insights that can be used to validate and normalize clients' experiences, especially those who may feel isolated, alone, and worried about the future of their well-being and familial relationships.

Overall, this book serves to fill the gaps of knowledge in working with donor families. This text centralizes years of research, advocacy, and interdisciplinary practice into one cohesive text that will be referenced for years to come. Mental health professionals trained in any modality can learn from and apply the information offered in this guide. Therapists who interface with donors, intended parents, donor-conceived people, and their extended families will find the information provided truly valuable, no matter their training or years of experience.

Breanna N. Beard, MA, Health Psychology Intern, Duke Fertility Center, Duke University Health System

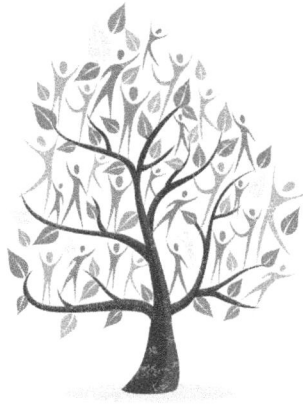

COUNSELING DONOR FAMILY MEMBERS

A Guide for Mental Health Professionals

Wendy Kramer

with Hilary Bertisch, PhD, ABPP

Counseling Donor Family Members: *A Guide for Mental Health Professionals*

Wendy Kramer, with Hilary Bertisch

This book first published 2022

Ethics International Press Ltd, UK

British Library Cataloguing in Publication Data

A catalogue record for this book is available from the British Library

Print Book ISBN: 978-1-80441-018-9

eBook ISBN: 978-1-80441-019-6

Table of Contents

Acknowledgements

A great deal of gratitude goes out to the thousands of egg and sperm donors, parents, and donor-conceived people who have shared their stories and experiences with me personally, via the Donor Sibling Registry, and through participation in our research studies. It is all of you, along with my son Ryan and his donor family, who made invaluable contributions to the ideas and advice contained in this guide.

Thanks to Leslie Gamble for helping us to birth the idea for this guide and for her early contributions, and thanks to Marcia Jacobs for her editing skills.

> *We should not be asking who this child belongs to,*
> *but who belongs to this child.*
> ~ Jim Gritter

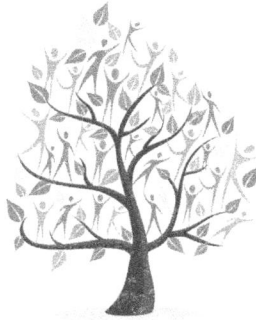

Preface

Infertility treatment has existed since the 1800s, beginning with the use of fresh sperm administered in a doctors' office, sometimes without the knowledge of the mother. We have come a very long way in terms of the technical and biological aspects of reproductive medicine, but in terms of the psychological and social aspects, an evolution of the practice has not come so quickly or easily.

In 1978, the first IVF baby was born and by the 1980s, and after a decline in the years surrounding the HIV/AIDS epidemic, the sperm donation industry also flourished. Increasing numbers of couples struggling with infertility, and later, single women (some single men), and LGBTQ+ couples turned to this industry to make their dreams of parenthood a reality.

Both adoption and assisted reproductive technologies are means of creating families outside of the traditional model of a biological mother and father also being the legal parents; both are alternatives for adults who are LGBTQ+, suffer from infertility, have a hereditary illness, or who do not have partners with whom they can procreate. Both also raise legal, ethical, and practical implications for everyone involved.[1] There is much to learn from the parallel world of adoption with regards to the importance of acknowledging a person's innate desire to learn about their close genetic relatives, ancestry, and medical backgrounds. Given the dramatic increase in the use of third-party reproduction in recent years combined with substantially greater access to genetic information through commercial DNA testing, it is therefore crucial for mental health professionals to have some background knowledge about how the gamete donation industry works and how donors, parents, and donor-conceived people's lives have been affected.

Over the years, there have been too many accounts from Donor Sibling Registry parents, donors, and donor-conceived people who were either not counseled at all, or who were counseled by therapists who did not seem well-versed or experienced in:

- The importance of early truth-telling about a child's conception story.

- The importance of acknowledging and honoring the right of all members of the donor family (i.e., the donor-conceived person, the donors, and the parents) to be curious about and search for genetic relatives.

- The trauma of finding the truth about one's donor-conception as an adult.

- The intricacies of donor family relationships.

- Or the potential complications and many joys of connecting with, and defining relationships with, newly discovered genetic families.

Given the considerable increase in the use of third-party reproductive technologies, it is increasingly likely that clinicians across a variety of mental health settings will encounter individuals who have been involved in this process in some capacity. In some cases, counseling may be indicated for donor-conceived people and their family members and also for donors and their family members. In other cases, these individuals may present for treatment for unrelated issues but have this kind of history that may surface. Many of these individuals may be new to treatment, and/or donor conception topics or concerns may arise unexpectedly during treatment for other issues. Clinicians must therefore be well-informed about all perspectives to provide compassionate and effective treatment.

Although it's imperative that parents and donors be adequately counseled *before* using a donor or donating, all too often, research demonstrates this is not the case. One 2013 published study of 1700 sperm recipients reported that 62% did not receive professional counseling before they embarked on conception using donor sperm, and neither did 72% of their partners.[2] Another 2009 study of 155 egg donors reported that only 37% of them felt as though they were properly educated and counseled about the potential curiosity of the children they were helping to create.[3] A 2013 study of 164 sperm donors found that 80% said they did not receive any education or counseling about the potential curiosities of donor-conceived people to know their genetic, ancestral and medical backgrounds.[4] Because facilities that sell the gametes have not incorporated this into their business models, all too often parents and donors have not been able to make fully-informed decisions about choices that will affect their own and their children's lives for decades to come.

There are currently few best practice rules, recommendations, or consolidated reporting systems in the United States, and no national oversight, regulations, or laws governing the gamete donor industry to protect all stakeholders. Although a few countries have recognized the needs of donor-conceived people, the US industry has remained relatively unchanged since those early days of secrecy and deception. This industry has, for the most part, had a limited response in considering the needs of donor-conceived people, donors, and parents when setting policy. Even though most donor-conceived people understand that they were deeply desired by their parents who went to great lengths to have them, many have been adversely medically and psychologically affected by the lack of regulation or oversight in the industry.

Mental health professionals are increasingly meeting with donor-conceived people and family members, necessitating knowledge and insight about their experiences and issues. The challenges of forming and redefining family for all donor family members considering and exploring their own or their child's new biological connections can be overwhelming. It's not uncommon for people to feel a sense of confusion or discomfort about their own conception story or their own or their family's boundaries when it comes to purchasing or selling gametes, issues surrounding disclosure, or reaching out to their own or their child's genetic relatives. Grappling with the depth and breadth, and the timing and speed with which they explore their own or their child's origins and expanding families can be challenging at times, but also deeply profound, rewarding, and joyous.

The qualitative and quantitative information presented in this guide comes from a broad and deep understanding based on decades of hearing from many thousands of donors and their families, parents, and donor-conceived people via the Donor Sibling Registry, both anecdotally and via dozens of published research studies conducted with research partners at major universities around the world. Some of the topics and issues have been presented with broad strokes, as they have been covered elsewhere, with more focus being placed on the issues that haven't been discussed enough in academia or elsewhere. Chapter 2 focuses on how the clinician can integrate this knowledge with theories and methods that they already have expertise in and use in practice.

The guide is intended to be a resource for mental health and medical professionals in any setting, and especially for those who are unfamiliar with the topic. It's a presentation of evolving ideas, recommendations, and talking points that can be used in counseling everyone in the donor family. Because each stakeholder is deeply connected to the others, understanding all viewpoints is important for a successful counseling experience with any of the stakeholders. Because the complete history of donor conception and all of its complexities are beyond the scope of this guide, there are references offered at the end of each section on the specific donor family member. A great place to start would be on the Donor Sibling Registry website (donorsiblingregistry.com) where dozens of published papers on egg donors, sperm donors, donor-conceived people, sperm recipients, egg donor parents, non-biological parents, and donor-grandparents can be found.

We hope to provide you with valuable information and appreciation for this increasingly visible and vocal population of donor family members that you will inevitably encounter in your practice.

Wendy Kramer

Wendy is Co-Founder and Director of the Donor Sibling Registry (DSR). The DSR was founded in 2000 with her donor-conceived son Ryan to assist individuals conceived as a result of sperm, egg, or embryo donation who are seeking to make mutually desired contact with others with whom they share genetic ties. With more than 80,000 members in 105 countries, the DSR has helped to connect more than 25,000 of them with their half-siblings and/or their biological parents, and Wendy has listened to and advised/consulted with thousands of these parents, donors, donor-conceived people, and other donor family members for more than two decades.

Wendy has conducted many research studies on all donor family members and is a co-author of the resulting peer-reviewed papers published in *Social Science and Medicine, Human Reproduction, Reproductive BioMedicine & Society, Facts, Views & Vision in OB/GYN, Reproductive BioMedicine Online (RBMOnline), Advances in Reproductive Sciences, Contemporary Perspectives in Family Research, Fertility and Sterility, The Journal of Family Issues, Children and Society, The Journal of Law and the Biosciences,* and more. She has contributed chapters to several books on donor conception and has reviewed abstracts for the American Society of Reproductive Medicine and has been a peer reviewer for the journals *Human Reproduction, RBMOnline, and Frontiers in Global Women's Health.*

Wendy was an Associate Producer for the 2011 *Emmy* nominated documentary *Sperm Donor* and on the 2013 MTV News & Docs, six-part docu-series called *Generation Cryo.* She co-wrote the book *Finding our Families: A First-of-Its-Kind Book for Donor-Conceived People and Their Families,*[5] wrote the children's book *Your Family: A Donor Kid's Story,*[6] and wrote *Donor Family Matters: My Story of*

Raising a Profoundly Gifted Donor-Conceived Child, Redefining Family, and Building the Donor Sibling Registry.[7]

Wendy was married when she gave birth to her son Ryan in 1990, and in 1991 began to raise him as an only parent. Ryan has connected with his biological father and knows of 23 half-siblings, so far. Wendy holds a B.A. in Communication Arts, has completed many postgraduate courses in counseling and psychology, is Mental Health First Aid certified, and is a *Psychology Today* contributor.

Hilary Bertisch

Hilary holds a Ph.D. in Clinical Psychology with a Board Certification in Clinical Neuropsychology. She is Assistant Professor in the Department of Psychiatry at the Donald and Barbara Zucker School of Medicine at Hofstra/Northwell in the New York City area and specializes in working with patients with psychosis and other brain-related conditions, many of which are characterized by trauma. Dr. Bertisch is also a late-discovery donor-conceived adult with lived experience of individuals who were conceived this way, particularly in the 1970s and 1980s. She is one of the very few known donor-conceived psychologists who has come forward to provide perspective on this topic to date and has served on the Board of Directors of the Donor Sibling Registry since 2019. Hilary authored the 2021 paper, *The Donor Conceived Adult: Implications Within Family, Medical, and Mental Healthcare Systems.*[8]

References

[1] Cahn, N. (2011). Old Lessons for a New World: Applying Adoption Research and Experience to Art, 24 *Journal of the American Academy of Matrimonial Lawyers*, 1.

[2] Sawyer, N., Blyth, E. Kramer, W. & Frith, L. (2013). A survey of 1700 women who formed their families using donor spermatozoa. *Reproductive Biomedicine Online, 27*, 436-447, doi: 10.1016/j.rbmo.2013.07.009

[3] Kramer, W., Schneider, J. & Schultz, N. (2009). US oocyte donors: A retrospective study of medical and psychosocial issues, *Human Reproduction, 24*, 3144–3149, https://doi.org/10.1093/humrep/dep309

[4] Daniels, K. R., Kramer, W. & Perez-y-Perez, M. V. (2012). Semen donors who are open to contact with their offspring: issues and implications for them and their families. *Reproductive BioMedicine Online, 25*, P670-677.m9.

[5] Kramer, W. & Cahn, N. (2013). *Finding Our Families: A First of Its Kind Book for Donor Conceived People and Their Families.* Penguin Publishing Group.

[6] Kramer, W. & Moore, J. (2018). *Your Family: A Donor Kid's Story.* Donor Sibling Registry, Colorado.

[7] Kramer, W. (2020). *Donor Family Matters: My Story of Raising a Profoundly Gifted Donor-Conceived Child, Redefining Family, and Building the Donor Sibling Registry.* Donor Sibling Registry, Colorado.

[8] Bertisch, H. & Kramer, W. (2021). The donor conceived adult: Implications within family, medical and mental healthcare systems. *Advance Medical and Clinical Research, 2*, 16-17.

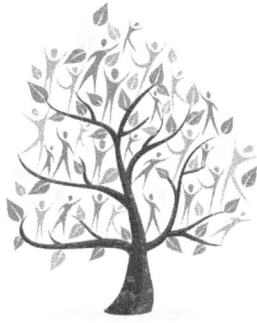

Chapter 1

Background Information on Donor Conception and Donor Families

Definitions

There can be inconsistency in the use of terms within the field of reproductive medicine. For example, the use of the term "donor" may imply one who provides selfless contribution, whereas most donors are paid for their sperm or eggs, except occasionally in the case of known donors. Accurate and honest terminology is an important factor in communication as it gives context to the content of our conversations. Knowledge of common definitions, terminology, and the vernacular is critical to optimizing communication with your donor family clients.

DNA Testing: Usually a commercial DNA test is taken to determine one's genetic relatives and ancestry via 23andme and/or Ancestry.com. For donor-conceived people (DCP), this type of genetic testing often turns up unexpected half-siblings and biological parents or their relatives. This is especially shocking for DCP who had no idea about their donor origins.

Donor: This is the person who sold their sperm or eggs. Most typically, but not always, this was for money. They are the biological but not the legal parent of the donor-conceived person, so they, therefore, have no parental rights or responsibilities. Donor-conceived people may refer to this person as their biological father/mother or genetic father/mother, or bio dad/mom, donor dad/mom, or simply as donor/father/mother. Donor-conceived people may use several of these terms depending who they're speaking with, and as they mature and define the relationship between themselves and the person who contributed around 50% of their DNA.

Donor-Conceived Person/People (DCP): The person who was created using the purchased gametes (or much more infrequently) the gametes donated by a family member or friend.

Donor Insemination (DI): Inserting purchased sperm into the recipient in order to create a pregnancy. This can be done at home or with the assistance of a doctor or nurse at a medical facility. Intrauterine insemination (IUI) is the most common procedure in which prepared sperm cells are placed directly into a woman's cervix or uterus to produce pregnancy.

Donor Sibling/Half-Sibling/Sibling/Dibling: These terms are interchangeable. These are the siblings created by parents using the same donor or from the donor's children that they themselves are raising. They share ~15%-30% of their DNA with each other. Donor-conceived people tend to prefer donor sibling, sibling, or half-sibling as some are offended by the term dibling, as they feel it minimizes the relationship.

Donor Sibling Registry (DSR): The Donor Sibling Registry is a 501(c)3 nonprofit organization founded in 2000 that connects, educates and supports egg and sperm donors (and their families), prospective parents, parents, and donor-conceived people. The DSR has facilitated mutual consent contact between more than 25,000 DCP and their half-siblings and/or their biological parents, the donors.

Gamete: The reproductive or genetic material, in the form of sperm or egg cell, that will contribute ~50% of a donor-conceived person's DNA.

Gamete Vendor: The clinic, sperm or egg bank, agency, doctor, or facility that purchases the gametes from the sperm or egg donor and then sells them (typically with a substantial mark-up), to the recipient family.

In Vitro Fertilization (IVF): IVF is a method of assisted reproduction that combines an egg with sperm in a laboratory dish. If the egg fertilizes and begins cell division, the resulting embryo is transferred into the woman's uterus where it will hopefully implant in the uterine lining and further develop. IVF is commonly used with purchased eggs and embryos.

Non-Biological/Social Parent: Parents who are raising a donor child but who have not contributed to the child's DNA. This includes the spouse or partner of a sperm recipient parent as well as the gestational recipient parent of an egg donor child. While epigenetic influences, like diet, alcohol, drugs, stress, and exposure to toxins can impact the fetus, the mother (or surrogate) who carries the child but who doesn't contribute the egg is not the genetic or biological parent. Parents using a donated embryo are the child's non-biological parents, similar to adoption. There is usually one non-biological parent in same-sex couples that purchase gametes. In most cases, these parents are also the legal parents.

Recipient: The intended parent(s) who purchases the gametes and who will raise the child.

Single Mother by Choice (SMC): Women began embracing single parenthood as a conscious choice in the late 70s. According to the singlemothersbychoice.org website, the term "single mothers by choice" first emerged in 1981 when NY psychotherapist, Jane Mattes founded her organization to provide support and resources to such moms. A SMC is a woman who chooses to be a single parent to a child/children without assistance or support from a partner. SMCs often build their families with gamete donation (using a known or unknown donor) and represent around 50% of the parents using donor sperm.

Reasons for seeking counseling: potential scenarios

Parents: Couples/people with infertility

- Infertility is painful. Clients experiencing male and female infertility may be feeling, loss, shame, disappointment, guilt, or anger. People with infertility might feel inadequate or like failures.

- Infertility may involve grief. Dealing with the stress of trying to conceive, many failed attempts at pregnancy, and/or pregnancy loss are common among people with infertility. A client presenting with depression may be experiencing unresolved grief or loss related to infertility struggles.

- Infertility is stressful. People with infertility and their partners often feel stress about the future. There can be worry about how using third-party reproduction will affect their partners and relationships. Additionally, infertility can cause financial stress because treatments and donor gametes can be very expensive.

- Infertility can cause fear. People considering infertility treatments and/or donor gametes are often scared about not being on the same page as their partner regarding the next steps in treatment and about the cost of those treatments. They may be afraid of the infertility treatments not working and never realizing their dreams of having children. Not knowing enough about donors and their medical histories can be unsettling. Additionally, there is fear of the unknown – not knowing about their future child's other genetic relatives or medical issues or about potential medical complications among those who carry donated eggs involving IVF procedures.

- Infertility can cause difficulties for egg (or embryo) recipients in understanding and accepting that although mothers who use an egg donor do carry and deliver a child and epigenetic influences are at play, they are not the genetic/biological parents because they do not contribute 50% of the child's DNA.

- Infertility can cause ambiguity when parents using donor gametes do not want to think about, plan for, or discuss issues and needs that their future donor-conceived children might have.

- Infertility can make some parents keep secrets. Infertile parents sometimes feel shame or other negative emotions that cause them to keep secret their experiences with infertility and/or using donor gametes. The secrets can last for decades and involve not talking about or allowing DCPs to feel comfortable expressing curiosity about or searching for donor relatives.

Parents: Single Mother by Choice (SMC) and LBGTQ single or couple recipients

Infertility can be a factor but donation, and usually disclosure, are a given in these situations. While some issues are unique to LGBTQ+ families and single parent families, these parents can share some common concerns.

- There may be concern about their child(ren) not having a father/mother or positive male/female role model.

- For SMCs, shame, embarrassment, guilt, and fear around nontraditional parenthood may arise. Additionally, there may be shame in not finding a spouse. Privacy is sometimes used as an excuse to cover up the secrecy/shame of why a donor was used.

- Financial stress can be a factor for SMCs who usually have no other income than their own paychecks, and struggle to make ends meet in a society that usually requires two incomes to achieve middle-income lives. When financial stress is present, it can negatively affect the day-to-day lives of these parents and their children because of the constant mental energy required to keep expenses low.

- For LGBTQ+ parents there may be stress or conflict in regards to whether to have a child and which partner will be genetically related to and/or carry the child.

- For LGBTQ+ parents there may be fears of legal parentage issues and fears by the non-biological parent that friends, family, and society will not view them as "real" parents.

- There can be difficulty with issues around the child's unknown genetic relatives, including a tendency to minimize or negate the importance of the genetic connection to the child's donor family.

- General discomfort with any conversations that include the donor or their contribution.

- Fear/shame about not being a "perfect parent" and that their child will like/love the donor (if searched for and located) more than them.

- Fear and/or hesitation when it comes to acknowledging the importance of connecting with the child's donor relatives.

- Fears around including new donor relatives into their own and their child's family circle.

Parents: Non-biological parents

Although some offspring indicate that their fathers were supportive and/or understanding regarding their curiosity about the donor, from the perspective of DCP, tensions related to donor conception are most prevalent in families headed by coupled heterosexuals.[1] This is true for families that use both eggs and sperm, including couples who have utilized dual donation (embryo or IVF using both donated egg and sperm). In heterosexual couples, there can be:

- Fear and/or embarrassment about others knowing about their infertility and use of a donor, and hesitance to acknowledge the donor's contribution.

- Struggling with the concept of not having biological connections with their child(ren), and/or being unable to fully bond with their child(ren).

- Fear that friends, family, and society will not view them as "real" parents.

Sperm or egg donors

Many gamete donors were told decades ago that their information would remain anonymous. In recent years anonymity has become almost impossible as DNA testing is now easily available. This can lead to:

- Embarrassment or shame about donation.

- Fear about disclosing to their partners that they not only donated gametes, but also have biological children as a result of their donations.

- Fear of marital/relationship problems related to donations and resulting children.

- Worrying about telling their children about their donations and potential half-siblings.

- Worrying about how to tell their parents that they may be grandparents to 10, 20, or even 200 DCPs.

- Feeling overwhelmed with a large group of progeny.

- Fear about opening themselves up to these new relationships, fear of rejection, fear of disrupting their families.

- Not having the emotional bandwidth to define these new relationships and not wanting contact.

- Fears about having rights, responsibilities or financial obligations for the children born from their donations.

- Confusion about their role and how to respond to requests for contact from parents and progeny, feelings of inadequacy, or being a disappointment to donor children (donors may not have been honest about or have successfully completed the studies that they indicated on their donor profiles).

- Wondering how to define these new relationships and possibly incorporate donor children into their family circles.

- Worry about sharing/updating medical information and learning about possible medical issues with progeny.

- Navigating the sometimes delicate line between privacy and secrecy. Protecting their family's privacy while removing the veil of secrecy between them and their progeny can be stressful as they try to balance the needs of everyone affected.

Donor's spouse (or partner)

- Anger at spouses/partners over secrecy around donation.

- Fear about what a relationship with progeny and/or the progeny's parents means for their marital relationship and for their children.

- Fear about the number of children that may enter their lives and what they might want/demand in terms of time and attention potentially taking away from the existing family.

- Disagreements with partners because they do not feel the same as them about contact.

- Difficulties in understanding and communicating their own comfort levels and privacy boundaries.

- Discomfort and difficulties in figuring out how to tell their children about half-siblings born from their spouse's/partner's donations.

- Excitement and/or intrigue about new and expanding genetic family.

Donor's child(ren) that they are raising, who find out that they have a half-sibling, or many, due to their parent's donation may feel:

- Confusion about how to define these new relationships: *what does this mean and who are these half-siblings to me*?

- Fear and frustration over changing family dynamics.

- Fear of losing the biological parent's attention and time.

DCP: Those whose conception stories have been shared with them since they were very young may feel or experience:

- Unrealistic or idealized expectations for their donor and/or experience subsequent disappointment.

- Overwhelmed at the number of half-siblings they may have.

- Struggles navigating relationships with siblings they've been raised with, and with new half-siblings whose experiences and feelings may be different from theirs.

- Frustration with the lack of available information about their donor and half-siblings, and with the gamete vendor that will not release what is known about their close genetic relatives.

- Ambiguous grief, loss, sadness, or a yearning to know the unknown biological parent or siblings.

- Rejection from attempted contact with the donor and/or half siblings (this is more likely to be a product of the donor's and half-siblings' own feelings and circumstances).

- No desire to connect with their half-siblings or biological parents. This can be complicated by having siblings they were raised with who do desire contact or half-siblings who desire or have already established contact with the donor.

- Attuned to the non-biological parent's discomfort with issues surrounding the donor, and know that these conversations are not encouraged.

- Challenges with re-defining family, setting boundaries, and navigating privacy/secrecy as they consider incorporating new relatives into their family circle.

- Fear of consanguinity and/or accidentally forming a romantic relationship with a person who has DNA from the same donor.

- Awareness that new genetic relatives are adding to a family, not taking away from it.

DCP: Those whose conception stories were kept from them may feel or experience:

- Anger at being lied to by the people they trust the most and finding out the truth as adults.

- Difficulty in figuring out how to talk to their parents about this new knowledge, if they found out on their own.

- Confusion, relief, curiosity, sadness.

- Disenfranchised grief, or feeling as though they are denied the right to grieve, do not have the social support essential to adapt to the loss, or feel deprived of social validation.

- The need to question their identity, normality, feelings, and to have to adapt to a new reality.

- Like their worlds and identities have been "turned upside down."

- The need for a deeper understanding and forgiveness for the parents who withheld the truth.

- Curiosity about their medical histories and new known, and still unknown, medical issues of close genetic family members.

- A desire to know more about their own biological identities, ancestry, and more about their close genetic relatives.

- Curiosity, interest, and even excitement about establishing relationships with biological parents (donors), their families, and with half-siblings.

- Difficulty knowing how to share their story with others who may not understand.

- Any or all of the items listed above for DCPs whose conceptions stories were not kept from them.

This story, shared by a donor conceived person, illustrates the possible, even inevitable, pain and trauma associated with having their conception story hidden from them:

Can you imagine living your entire life basically a lie of who your father was? Looking back I always knew something wasn't right. I am not going to blame my parents because they were told by the doctors to never tell; however, I still feel it was best to be HONEST. It would have truly shaped me in a different way. They are now saying tell your children AS EARLY AS POSSIBLE because of the psychological effects. Was it traumatic? You bet!!! Imagine looking in the mirror and trying to figure out who you are again? I was angry, hurt, traumatized, broken, lost, and it was a long grieving and healing process. Do I still believe my parents loved me? Absolutely. Did I still believe my parents believed they were doing the best for me? Yes, absolutely. However, this was not an easy walk. Now, I am choosing not to hide my IDENTITY of WHO I AM. I will not keep it a secret and follow the same path and be filled with shame. Just like when we know someone was adopted it is very similar in that way. We go through the same psychological factors as when someone doesn't find out they are adopted until later in life.

So here I am sharing my story. I came into a family of almost 20 siblings that we know of, and an Aunt who is lovingly involved in our lives. Unfortunately, the donor does not want involvement but he is a doctor and is healthy and in great shape (he competes in competitions). I have met 2 siblings so far in person. We have Skype meetings and yearly group meetups, although I am not quite ready for that yet. ;) I have finally found WHY I do what I do and can see qualities that I share with the other siblings. It has been a crazy journey but this is WHO I AM and where I came from. I hope you will be understanding with me opening up as well as be compassionate — and if you have a story to tell, please don't hold back. It could change someone's life.

General themes that affect all stakeholders

Disclosure: why should I tell my child that they are donor-conceived?

Some parents are reluctant to tell their children that they were conceived with donor gametes. In the past, it was strongly advised by the physicians not to tell and presently, some may feel that openness jeopardizes the gamete vendor industry as it allows access to relationships that may be unwanted, especially by the donors. This information is therefore portrayed as "private" or "confidential." Married, heterosexual couples are more likely to feel this way than either single women or same-sex couples who use donor sperm. In many cases, heterosexual couples have not shared the information with any close friends or family.

Parents who believe their children deserve to know their genetic origins tend to frame the issue in terms of "honesty" versus "secrecy." In order to have mutual trust, these parents expect honesty from their children and at the same time feel that they owe their children the same. They value openness in the family and believe that secrets can be dangerous and uncontrollable. For example, in cases where there are some other people who do know the circumstances of a child's conception, there is always the risk of unplanned and traumatic disclosure by someone besides the parent.

Children benefit from being told about the circumstances of their conception for three primary reasons: 1) they have a right to know their genetic origins, 2) withheld information can damage trust between family members, 3) secrecy can also lead to feelings of inadequacy, shame and/or of inferiority in DCP, because children often blame themselves for family problems, and DCPs can be left to wonder why the truth was withheld from them – *was it because there is something wrong with me?*

Some donor-conceived people who had not yet been told that they were donor-conceived reported that they already felt different within their families, based on either physical characteristics or personality, but lacked the facts to substantiate their strong feelings. Even without being told, children are often attuned to hidden clues from the family. In the studies that have been completed with donor-conceived people, many have reported a powerful sense that valuable information was being withheld from them.[1]

The early 2000s brought about the ability for parents to make mutual consent contact with their child's half-siblings and donors through the DSR and that raised new issues about disclosure. Parents who had always told their children that they were donor-conceived, now also needed to decide when and how to tell their children about new relatives that had been found.

Talking honestly, even to very young children, and modeling these conversations so that children can feel confident about sharing their origin stories, especially when the parent isn't present, is vital. The importance of early disclosure of the child's origin story cannot be stressed enough. Parents can start this dialogue when their children are preverbal so that it becomes an integrated part of a donor child's identity. As with many conversations with young children, they might not comprehend the depth and breadth of all the concepts, but they will gradually absorb the facts as they mature. Creating these cornerstone conversations to build upon as a child matures is essential.

Different perceptions of the donor: nature and nurture

To some parents, a donated egg or sperm might seem like just a donated cell or a piece of genetic material, as this is how the gamete vendors often frame gamete donation. But to a DCP, it's the origin of approximately 50% of their DNA: one half of their identity, ancestry, physical attributes, and medical/psychological origins. Many DCP, just like those who are adopted (many of whom have great relationships with their parents), often feel a deep-seated need to know their genetic relatives, or at the very least know about them, to better understand themselves. Donors also often wonder about the children that were created as a result of their donations. They wonder if they look like them, share any traits, and if they are healthy and happy.

The reality is that we're all a unique and wonderful blend of nature *and* nurture. The people that raise us and love us, our families, our communities, our experiences, and the two people that gave us our DNA blueprint, all factor into who we become as adults.

General seeking/searching/finding themes:

- Curiosity. *Who are my (or my child's)* close genetic relatives?

- DCP wondering about their identity, ancestry, and medical backgrounds.

- Ethical and/or legal dilemmas; for example, some parents are afraid of breaching the anonymity agreement they signed with the gamete vendor.

- Psychological/medical concerns: sharing one's own issues and/or finding out that close genetic relatives have issues that may be genetic in nature.

- The fear of rejection.

- The excitement of searching for, and finding, new family.

- The challenge of defining new genetic relationships.

- Fear of incorporating new people into their family and upsetting the family balance.

- Fear of betraying the non-biological parent.

- Fear of parents or other relatives not being supportive.

- Fear of not finding any information about their own or their child's donor origins or close genetic family.

- Maneuvering through their own and other family members' privacy and secrecy boundaries.

Re-defining family

Family can no longer be defined in the simple black-and-white terms that have been used in the past in this country, and in many countries around the world. More and more donor families are expanding the traditional family to include some kind of relationship with half-siblings, the donor, and even with the donor's family. For many decades donor anonymity was mandated and expected, but now it has become an antiquated notion with many negative repercussions. Since 2000 almost 30,000 DCP have connected with half-siblings and/or genetic parents on the DSR, and many thousands more have connected via commercial DNA testing companies. Breaking down the walls of anonymity has precipitated new and evolving ideas about how we now define family. As helping professionals counselors can examine our own experiences of family and also think about expanding our definitions of family.

Problems created and perpetuated by the gamete vendors

The fertility industry is largely unregulated in the United States.[2] They are a for-profit industry and have historically valued their interests and the interests of the donors and the parents over the interests of donor-conceived people. This model provides their financial foundation. As DNA testing and resources such as the DSR have become increasingly available to the donor family community, however, the legacy of secrecy is no longer realistic, and the ethics of the practice have been increasingly questioned. Many have experienced the reproductive medicine industry promising and promoting secrecy and perpetuating deceptive practices.

It is vital that helping professionals understand the gaps in information that the families are still told and the problems that may result later on.

What do we mean by this?

Secrecy

The earliest known documentation on donor insemination is from 1884 with a Quaker family presenting with male-factor infertility at Jefferson Medical College in Philadelphia. The wife was anesthetized and unaware that she was inseminated with donor sperm from a medical student; the husband provided consent and the procedure was successful. Similar procedures continued off the record in doctor's offices for many decades.[3,4]

Although the idea of openness has increased relative to the procedures uniformly implemented in the past, gamete vendors and doctors continue to encourage secrecy, thinly veiled as privacy, and promoted as in the best interests of all donor family members. People are still routinely advised not to disclose to friends, family, or even the child about the use of donated gametes. Secrecy often implies shame, and this shame is often transmitted to the child as shame about their donor conception. Additionally, secrecy is also illustrated in a gamete vendor's lack of transparency in regard to record keeping, sharing medical information longitudinally, medical follow-ups, information on the children born from donors, and other vital information. Because DCP's who are aware of their status have little opportunity to talk about it to others who understand, they may not have the language to speak about their experience and thus continue to keep it secret.

This secrecy can be difficult for DCP to cope with as they try to integrate the truth about their conception into their self-identities. From a donor-conceived person:

I was conceived by a donor egg in 1988. My mom says she does not remember any of the basic information about the egg donor (ethnicity, medical history, etc.). I have called the clinic where I was conceived multiple times, left messages and never gotten a response back. The only information

I have is the serial number of the petri dish I was made in, because the clinic gave my mom the petri dish as a souvenir. I am G**80.

I got that number tattooed on the back of my neck. I guess it was my way of trying to re-establish control and ownership of my own body after I had been told I had no legal rights (seeing as I was the product, and not one of the people involved) to my own genetic history and information.

I love my mom and her family, but it has always been extremely obvious that I do not share genetic material with them; aside from physical appearance, we have absolutely nothing in common in terms of shared interests, aptitudes, dislikes, taste, or personal traits. We are polar opposites to a comical degree.

Legal Fears

One sperm bank has gone as far as threatening (via a failed legal attempt) a parent who had tested their child's DNA and reached out to close relatives on DNA websites, claiming that DNA testing a donor-conceived child is breaking the privacy agreement that the parent signed with the sperm bank.[5] Parents can therefore be fearful of legal repercussions from the gamete vendors. All stakeholders can make mutual consent contact, as there are no laws or regulations prohibiting parents from reaching out to their donors, and donor-conceived people never signed an agreement prohibiting them from reaching out to their biological parent and/or their family. In an attempt to keep parents and DCP from donors, gamete vendors sometimes perpetuate these misconceptions by including threatening legal verbiage in their agreements.

In further attempts to keep donors and parents from connecting with each other, it's common for the gamete brokers to create the perception about parents who will want donors to be financially responsible, and donors who will want to exert parental rights over the child. Both fallacies only serve to perpetuate the industry's desire for secrecy. Parents don't look to the donors to be financially responsible for their children. Donors who donate via gamete vendors are not legal parents and therefore have no legal rights or responsibilities and do not desire to usurp parents or actively parent the children they help to create.

Deception

There is a need for reform in the gamete vendor industry so that practices can become more transparent, uniform, consistent, and ethical. There are many reports of recipients receiving gametes from someone other than the donor they contracted to receive, including from doctors, from a donor with more than 100 or 200+ donor children, and from those with a medical and/or psychological disease that was known yet undisclosed and hidden from potential recipients.[2,6-10] Even when a known verified genetically linked disease is later reported by the donor or recipients, the gamete vendors have oftentimes failed to pull remaining vials out of circulation, thereby allowing that genetic material to be passed on to even more offspring. These gamete vendors routinely fail to notify recipients about these medical issues, exacerbating a delay in screenings, diagnosis, and treatment of sometimes life-altering conditions.

Sperm and egg facilities that promise to get regular or yearly updated medical information from donors rarely follow through. In a 2012 study of 164 donors, 85% of 164 surveyed sperm donors and 97% of 155 egg donors surveyed in 2009 have never been contacted by their gamete vendor for a medical update, while 23% of the sperm donors and 31% of those egg donors felt that they, or a close family member, had medical/genetic issues that would be important to share with families.[11,12] New research, conducted in 2021 with 345 egg donors, showed that in eleven years, practices have remained similar: more than 94% were never contacted for a medical update, while 25% indicated that they did have a medical issue that would be important to share with families. To make matters worse, 62% with a medical issue indicated that their clinic was dismissive when they tried to report the medical issue.[13]

DNA = Donors Not Anonymous

Gamete vendors still recruit donors with promises of anonymity and every gamete sold is sold as anonymous, be it for 18 years, or forever. This, along with gamete vendors' failure to verify what the donor voluntarily reports, has led to misrepresentation of areas including criminal history, educational attainment, mental illness, and genetic disease. They promise/mandate anonymity to the donor without any information about what the future may hold and require recipients to promise never to try to seek out the donor for any reason. In the past, that was fairly easy to maintain. Even with a growing population of donor-conceived people fighting for their rights to their own medical and genealogy data, the secret was pretty safe until 2005, when the first donor-conceived person found his donor via DNA testing.[14]

Until the late 1970s families were given little to no information about the donor. Since the advent of sperm banks in the late 1970s and early 1980s, most parents have been given non-identifying facts about the person who would contribute 50% of their child's genes, along with a donor number/ID. Since 2000 these donor numbers/IDs have made it possible for more than 25,000 donor-conceived people to connect with their half-siblings and donors on the Donor Sibling Registry.

With the introduction of commercially available DNA testing (*Family Tree DNA* in 2004, *23andme* 2007, *Ancestry.com* in 2012, and others like *MyHeritage*), the assurance of anonymity is no longer possible; it has been estimated that 90% of Americans of European descent are now identifiable from their DNA, even without ever having taken a DNA test themselves.[15] Many DCP born from the 1940s through the 1980s who didn't have the luxury of a donor number are now easily connecting with half-siblings and biological parents (and their families) via the DNA websites.

Why is this important?

- **Ancestry**: Conduct any Google search for donor-conceived people and you will quickly see what a significant number of DCP have to say about anonymity. Research also tells us that a large percentage of DCP desire to know about their other biological parent, the donor.[1] Many feel that they did not agree to any secrecy, and, just like everyone else, feel that they should have the right to know about their genetic identity, ancestry, and who their first-degree relatives are.

- **Medical History**: It's not uncommon to hear about DCP or their parents who have found out that very little of what they were told about a donor turned out to be true. A family medical history and medical updates are important throughout our lives for pre-screening and preventative care. A donor's profile only includes a self-reported snapshot of one day in the life of a healthy young person, which can be problematic as many diseases are adult-onset. It can be crucial for both the DCP and the donor to share and update information with each other since an inherited physical and mental disease that happens in the donor (or his children) could later affect the DCP and vice-versa.

- **Family Secrets:** We, as helping professionals, should be well versed in the dangers and toxicity of family secrets. From substance abuse to domestic violence to the stigma of mental health, research abounds about the damage that family secrets and deception create and their role in maladaptive family dynamics. The cognitive dissonance created by having a helping professional advise families to keep such a basic truth from their loved ones, and worse, from the child(ren) created, can be problematic and serve to increase the problems within the family. Many families say they knew this advice seemed wrong.

- **Impact of Large Donor Cohorts**: Another important issue that might surface is how having 50, 100, or more than 200 half-siblings or donor children might affect DCP and donors. When the Donor Sibling Registry was first established in 2000, most members thought that each donor might have a handful of offspring, as many were told by the sperm banks that each donor would have no more than ten kids. (There are no known reports of half sibling groups of more than around a dozen children from egg donors.) As time went on, families who had children later in the 1990s and into the 2000s were told no more than twenty children or twenty families, sometimes in a geographic area. Over the years, as donor families started connecting with each other, some once-small half-sibling groups have grown from 10 or 20 into 50 and then 100 and now more than 225. It's abundantly clear that the limits and numbers given by the sperm banks were and still are inaccurate. They can't enforce limits until they have an accurate accounting of all the children born for any one donor, which no sperm bank has.

There are many medical and psychosocial reasons why 50 or more than 200 kids from one donor may be problematic:

- If a donor has a heritable genetic medical issue, it could be passed along to dozens of his biological children. If a donor-conceived person doesn't know all of their half-siblings, they could be missing out on sharing their own medical information and learning about medical information from others. There may be genetic issues that would warrant proper screenings, monitoring, or preventative medicine.

- A donor with dozens or hundreds of donor children is less likely to connect with those kids later on, just because of the sheer number. DCP in these large groups who desire contact with their biological parent may never get it, just because the sperm bank was careless.

- Although sperm banks try to minimize the possibility of random meetings, this is not an uncommon experience. With that many offspring, meetings are much more likely. Consanguinity is a concern.

- Many DCP report feeling like they are part of a "herd" of offspring or like a commodity, a product that was sold and bought.

References

[1] Beeson, D., Kramer, W. & Jennings, P. K. (2011). Offspring searching for their sperm donors: how family type shapes the process. *Human Reproduction*, 26, 2415–2424, doi: https://doi.org/10.1093/humrep/der202

[2] America's love of free markets extends to its fertility clinics. *The Economist*, March, 2021.

[3] Kramer. W. (January 2022). A brief history of donor conception. *Huffpost.com*

[4] Bertisch, H. & Kramer, W. (2021). The donor conceived adult: Implications within family, medical and mental healthcare systems. *Advance Medical and Clinical Research*, 2, 16-17.

[5] Teuscher v. CCB-NWB, LLC, NO: 2:19-CV-0204-TOR (E.D. Wash. Oct. 22, 2019). https://casetext.com/case/teuscher-v-ccb-nwb-llc

[6] Glover, C. (May, 2020). To beat COVID-19 boredom this only child is connecting with multiple newly discovered half-siblings. *CBS News*.

[7] Denney, A. (May 10, 2019). Manhattan sperm bank didn't properly screen for genetic diseases: suit. *New York Post*.

[8] Mroz, J. (September, 2011). One Sperm Donor, 150 Offspring. *The New York Times*.

[9] Mroz, J. (May, 2012) In Sperm Banks, a Matrix of Untested Genetic Disease, *The New York Times*.

[10] Marcus, A. D. (January 2, 2022). A Grieving Family Wonders: What if They Had Known the Medical History of Sperm Donor 1558? *The Wall Street Journal*.

[11] Daniels, K. R. Kramer, W. & Perez-y-Perez, M. V. (2012). Semen donors who are open to contact with their offspring: issues and implications for them and their families. *Reproductive BioMedicine Online*, 25, P670-677.m9o.

[12] Kramer, W., Schneider, J. & Schultz, N. (2009). US oocyte donors: a retrospective study of medical and psychosocial issues. *Human Reproduction*, 12, 3144-3149. doi: 10.1093/humrep/dep309

[13] Adlam, K., Koenig, M. D., Patil, C., Salih, S., Steffen, A., Kramer, W. & Hershberger, P. E. (2021). The disclosure experiences of egg donors across the lifespan. Poster accepted to the annual conference of the *Midwest Nursing Research Society* (MNRS).

[14] Motluck, A. (November 3, 2005). Anonymous sperm donor traced on internet. *NewScientist.com*

[15] Murphy, H. (October 11, 2018). Most White Americans' DNA Can Be Identified Through Genealogy Databases. *New York Times*.

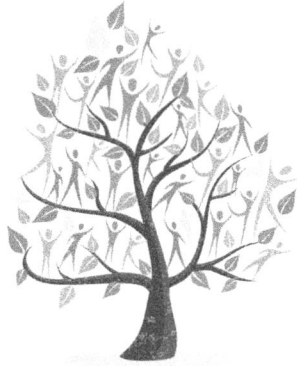

Chapter 2

Standard Assessment

Assess and formulate the client's experience

As in working with any new client, the goals of the initial phase of treatment are to clarify your client's experience and in doing so, help them in 1) gaining a more complete understanding of their own thoughts and feelings, 2) verbalizing them, 3) processing them, 4) accepting them, 5) empowering the client, and 6) teaching them that they are not alone. This work generally translates across clients with many kinds of presenting problems, and in cases of individuals who have been directly involved in assisted reproduction, it is only once they identify and work through their feelings can they best move forward with the next action steps.

Assessment & formulation of the issues

- First, be confident. The client in front of you may be experiencing trauma and/or a difficult set of decisions, and although you may be less experienced with this particular set of issues, you may have worked with variations of the same underlying themes before. Most likely, you have experience in helping clients work through unfamiliar situations, diagnoses, and traumas, even if you are not an expert in each of these specific areas. Given the relative newness of this area, there are very few experts in this field to date. The general principles and tools for initial assessment and formulation are the same as they would be for clients presenting with a range of other problems.

- In terms of assessment of the problem, follow standard interview procedures. Identify the chief issues and how the client experiences them (using both their verbal and non-verbal cues), assess your own feelings (including those of insecurity in handling a new situation like this), and begin to establish rapport. When possible, speak in the client's own language[1,2] and refer to Chapter 1 of this guide for a list of definitions of terms that may be unfamiliar to you.

- Begin your formulation for treatment using the theoretical frameworks you already know. What are the mechanisms of change that you are already most familiar with? As a clinician, have you found it to be more helpful to clarify the client's thoughts surrounding his/her circumstances (i.e., as in a cognitive-behavioral approach) or do you generally start by understanding the feelings underlying them? Research has shown that in general psychotherapy samples, the relationship with the psychotherapist is more important than the modality used for treatment in predicting outcome,[3] and that some aspects of therapy are common to all modalities.[4] Just as your preferred approach may work well with a client with any other presenting problem, it may therefore work well here. Regardless of the overt presenting problem, undoubtedly the thoughts and feelings underlying the experience are ones that you've worked with in other situations before. Remember that it is also acceptable to learn from your client.

- As in working with any client, tailor your formulation and treatment according to the individual sitting in front of you.[5] Understand the client's perception of the issue within the context of his/her personality,[4] generation, family system, environment, and culture. Validate his or her experience as indicated within the context of these frameworks. As always, identify the client's strengths as a means "to broaden client perspectives and create hope and motivation, to create positive meanings through reframing and metaphors.....and to amplify strengths through encouragement and exception finding."[6] Create a collaboration and discover their experiences with them.

Examining your own feelings and impressions throughout

"It is often the assessment of one's own affect [impression] that allows [the psychotherapist] to make a critical diagnostic inference."[7] In other words, psychotherapists are constantly using our own reactions to our clients to develop our formulations and to inform treatment. This may be particularly relevant to thoughts and feelings that the client may not yet be able to verbalize. For instance, in the case of the DCP, do you feel frustrated or overwhelmed when you are with this client? What are the implications of this for how this individual may actually be feeling? How may this information assist you in guiding the person to better put words to and ultimately better accept his/her experience in order to later determine how to best respond?

Knowing your limits, seeking additional resources, and when to refer out

Any competent psychotherapist should be aware of his or her own limits of practice with any client and the same is true in working with a client who is presenting with issues related to donor conception. It is important to decipher when supplemental resources, reading, consultation, and/or supervision may assist you in working with an individual facing these challenges, versus when additional factors and/or feelings may interfere with your own ability to assist the client through the first phase of treatment in an objective, supportive manner. It has been well-recognized that "psychotherapists need not offer all services to all clients." In the event that this client is not a fit for your practice, it is our professional obligation to "consider a judicious referral to a colleague who can offer the relationship stance (or treatment method) indicated in [this] particular case."[5]

Translation of general therapy concepts to all donor family members

- **Non-judgmental listening:** Many people feel better by telling their stories and receiving acknowledgment for their experience and the thoughts and feelings they're having.

- **Acknowledging and validating:** Everything your client is feeling is appropriate, normal, and to be expected.

- **They are not alone:** Many people have walked this path before your client. There is so much we've learned from those who have already successfully made the journey. It's important to have patience and know that there is plenty of information and support available.

- **Empowerment**: It's not uncommon for people to feel a sense of confusion or discomfort about their own conception story or their own or their family's boundaries when it comes to purchasing or selling gametes, issues surrounding disclosure, or reaching out to their own or their child's genetic relatives. Parents, donors, and DCP should all know that they are in control of their own process as they work through associated fears, hesitations, feelings, and emotions. It is important to remind them that they are not powerless and do have control of the depth and breadth as well as the timing and speed with which they make their connections as they explore their own feelings, emotions, origins, and expanding families.

References

[1] Morrison, J. (1995). Openings and Introductions. In Morrison, J. *The First Interview: Revised for DSM-IV* (pp 7-13). The Guilford Press, New York, NY.

[2] Morrison, J. (1995). Chief Complaint and Free Speech. In Morrison, J. *The First Interview: Revised for DSM-IV* (pp 14-22). The Guilford Press, New York, NY.

[3] Saxon, D., Frick, N. & Barkham, M. (2017). The relationship between therapist effects and therapy delivery factors: Therapy modality, dosage, and non-completion. *Administration and Policy in Mental Health and Mental Health Services*, 44, 705–715. https://doi.org/10.1007/s10488-016-0750-5

[4] Gurman, A. S. & Messer, S. B. (1995). Essential Psychotherapies: An Orienting Framework. In Gurman A. S. and Messer, S. B. *Essential Psychotherapies: Theory and Practice* (pp 1-11). The Guilford Press, New York, NY.

[5] Norcross, J. C. & Wampold, B. E. (2011). What works for whom: Tailoring psychotherapy to the person. *Journal of Clinical Psychology: In Session*, 67, 127–132.

[6] Scheel, M. J., Davis, C. K. & Henderson, J. D. (2012). Therapist use of client strengths: A qualitative study of positive processes. *The Counseling Psychologist*, 1-36, v doi: 10.1177/0011000012439427

[7] McWilliams, N. (1999). Assessing Affects. In McWilliams, N. *Psychoanalytic Case Formulation* (pp 102-121). The Guilford Press, New York, NY.

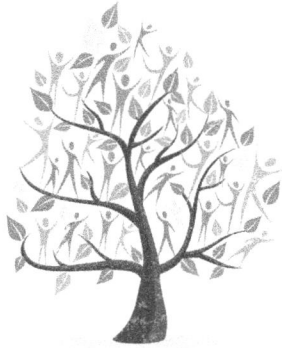

Chapter 3

Prospective Parents

Exploration of thoughts and feelings of prospective parents

It is important to understand themes that commonly arise with people thinking about using donated gametes. Given the historical secrecy surrounding donor conception, there was little empirical literature in the area until the past few decades, and this area of study continues to evolve.

Both available research and decades of anecdotal accounts suggest themes in the experience of parents of adult DCP that prospective parents should be aware of when making important decisions and planning for their future child.[1]

Questions and topics to explore with the prospective parent client:

- What are the clients' beliefs about fertility and infertility?

- How does your client define "family"?

- Grief over infertility and/or pregnancy loss (sometimes multiple), and the impact that will have on their future children.

- Loss of the fantasy of the "perfect family."

- For prospective parents who will have no genetic connection with their children, loss of the hope for a genetic link to their child, or their child being genetically connected to only one parent in a couple.

- Deciding what the use of donor gametes will mean to them, their family, and their future child.

- Financial concerns. Donor conception can be very expensive, especially for single mothers by choice. These moms should have a financial plan that includes ways to cover conception expenses, medical expenses resulting from pregnancy and birth, and living expenses during a maternity leave from employment.

- Does the prospective parent have a strong social support network? Choosing donor conception is rarely an easy journey. Having close friends and family members available to support prospective parents during the journey is essential, as is having this social network after a child is born.

- Emotional protection of the non-biological parent.

- Privacy and the desire to hide the shame of infertility or of not having a partner.

- Choosing a donor: not knowing enough about what they look like or what kind of person they are, and considering which donor characteristics are most important to them and which ones might be genetic in nature, e.g., high intelligence or kindness and empathy.

- Will they be okay with carrying (or having their partner carry) the baby of someone unknown to them?

- Worry that their children won't look like them.

- Their perceptions about how their family/community/society will view them as parents if people know their child's conception story.

- Concern over unknown or unreported medical issues that could be passed to their future child.

- The desire to protect themselves behind the (false) screen of anonymity with other families who used the same donor or with the donor.

- How and when to disclose to the child, family, and others.

- Issues regarding holding family "secrets" and the damage that they can have on relationships, families, and especially on DCP.

- The legal and emotional issues that might result from using a known donor, (a friend, family member, or stranger found via social media).

- Fears about not being able to connect with and love the child. It is crucial that this fear be adequately addressed before deciding to utilize donor conception.

Understanding the needs of Donor-Conceived People

Based on available research and a wealth of experience we believe that DCP, like everyone else, should have the right:

- To fully know their origin stories.

- To know about their ancestry, because part of knowing who you are is knowing who and where you come from.

- To know about their close genetic relatives: half-siblings, biological parents, biological grandparents, etc.

- To have their full medical history to ensure proper preventative evaluation, screenings, and treatments.

- To have parents willing to be honest and open, and to discuss all donor issues.

- To have the freedom to explore their genetic identity and connections without any guilt or fear of hurting their parents.

It is important to understand the challenges with using either an "open" (sometimes called "open identity" or "willing-to-be known") or an anonymous donor. An "open" donor is one who agrees to be contacted by any children resulting from their gametes, once they are 18. However, there are no guarantees that "open" donors will be found or will be willing to make contact, so it is important to discuss realistic expectations. Because anonymity is no longer possible, parents of minors can accept or even embrace the idea of connecting with their child's unknown genetic parent and likely, a host of half-siblings via the Donor Sibling Registry or via the DNA/ancestry companies.

Recommendations for prospective parents

Just give me a baby, I'll worry about everything else later! Many prospective parents are coming from a place of desperation, afraid they won't ever be able to have the child they so desperately desire. This can keep them from doing their due diligence to fully educate themselves and to fully consider the ramifications of using donated gametes. Prospective parents should be reminded that the decisions they make today in choosing a gamete vendor, choosing a donor, selecting an "anonymous" vs. an "open" donation, etc., can affect their future child for decades to come. Helping clients realize the magnitude of these decisions and the importance of pacing themselves so they can make educated and informed choices is vital.

- Encourage your client to talk with their current support system about their plans. This can be a joyful event with no shame around it. The more open they are now, the easier it will be to be open and honest after a child is born. Fewer family secrets are the foundation for this.

- Help your client also build support systems around donor conception. Encourage them to seek out other parents of DCP, especially parents of older DCP. These others can become a source of information and encouragement along their journey. Encourage them to explore the Donor Sibling Registry and read the success stories, testimonials, research, and the wealth of information provided. Hearing advice from others who have walked the path before them can be incredibly helpful.

- It is important for prospective parents to know the importance of early conception story disclosure and that they will be modeling, with both words and tone, conversations about donor conception for their very young children. They can prepare for these conversations. It's important for these parents to understand that the more their children see them speak confidently with family, friends, teachers, acquaintances, and even strangers, the more comfortable their children will feel, and the more comfortable they will feel when leaving their kids at school or at a birthday party. Parents can feel confident that any playground questions won't rattle their child, as their child will be self-assured about explaining and sharing their own origin story.

- Parents should be aware that donor-conceived people are quite often very curious about their ancestry, medical backgrounds, and close genetic family. It's important for parents to acknowledge that their kids will most likely think about and want to talk about their unknown genetic relatives. Talking through a prospective parent's hesitations and having an understanding of the benefits of honoring their child's curiosities and desires to connect with their genetic relatives is imperative.

- It's now very common for same-sex male couples and heterosexual couples utilizing egg donation to join the DSR to connect with their egg donor right from pregnancy/birth. This allows the parents and the donor to establish contact and decide for themselves the depth, breadth, and speed with how they communicate and how to define their relationships. These connections allow DCP to grow up having access to their genetic parent and possible half-siblings.

Now that you have gathered the initial information about your client and their experience of considering gamete donation to build their family, just as with any client presenting with a new area of focus, it is important to educate yourself on this topic. Reading this guide is a great start.

> *To the extent prospective parents choose donor conception over adoption, it is because they prefer to raise a biologically related child. If the desire for a biological connection is strong enough to make adults choose donor conception over adoption, then it is the ultimate double standard to imagine that the desire for a biological connection will not be felt just as strongly by the donor-conceived person. I believe our thinking on this issue has been distorted by a medical model that sees infertility as a problem to which the creation of a baby is the solution. People need to understand that donor conception does not create a 'baby.' It creates a human being who is forced to live with the lifelong consequences of choices made by the adults involved in their creation.* **-DCP**

> *Donor conception enables women to have a child with a biological connection (versus adoption) yet severs that same connection between the offspring and the paternal family. In other words, treating one person's loss (infertility) potentially creates loss in someone else (the donor offspring).* **-DCP**

> *We know our families love us and wanted us enough to go to extraordinary measures to have us, but who wants to start a book on chapter 2? I want Chapter 1, the Introduction and the Prologue as well!* **-DCP**

References

[1] Blyth, E., Kramer, W. & Schneider, J. (2013). Perspectives, experiences, and choices of parents of children conceived following oocyte donation. *Reproductive Biomedicine Online*, 6, 179-88. doi: 10.1016/j.rbmo.2012.10.013.

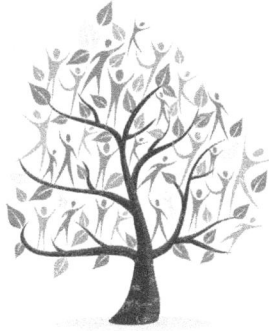

Chapter 4

Donor-Conceived People (DCP)

Exploration of thoughts and feelings of the donor-conceived person (DCP)

It is important to understand themes that commonly arise with DCP. Given the historical secrecy surrounding donor conception, there was little empirical literature in the area until the past few decades, and this area of study continues to evolve. Both available research and decades of anecdotal accounts do suggest themes in the experiences of donor-conceived people that you may expect to be reported in the context of assessment and treatment sessions, which are listed below.[1,2]

Common themes reported by DCP, even if they are seeking counseling for other reasons:

- Curiosity about, and establishing relationships with, donors, their families, and/or with half-siblings,[3] and frustration with a lack of available information, specifically with the gamete vendor who will not release what is known about their close genetic relatives.[4]

- Curiosity about medical history and about new and still unknown medical issues of close genetic family members.[5,6]

- Interest in contacting the donor. The vast majority of offspring in all types of families desire contact with their donor; however, comfort in expressing curiosity regarding one's donor may be lowest in dual-parent heterosexual families, with about one-quarter reporting an inability to discuss their origins with their social father.[1]

- Lack of male role models. For DCP with SMC or LGBTQ+ parents who have grown up knowing about their donor status, growing up without a father or sufficient male role models might present in treatment. One large study reported that 37.1% of DCP with LGBTQ+ parents indicated that they had felt something missing from not being parented by a male figure.[7]

- Navigating relationships with half-siblings whose experiences and feelings may be different from theirs.

- The rejection or perceived rejection from attempted contact with the donor. This rejection is more likely to be a product of the donor's own feelings and circumstances rather than your client's.

- The rejection or perceived rejection from half-siblings.

- Challenges with redefining family: setting boundaries and navigating privacy/secrecy as they consider incorporating new relatives into their family circle.

- Understanding that new genetic relatives are adding to a family, not taking away from it.

- Incorporating a large number of half-siblings into their lives[8,9] as discovering dozens, or more than 100, is no longer uncommon.

- The legal and emotional issues that might result if they were conceived using a known donor, (a friend, family member, or stranger found by their parents via social media).

For DCP whose conception stories were not shared with them as children, having information withheld by the people they trust the most and finding out the truth as adults can be a traumatic experience, causing feelings of having their worlds and identities being turned upside down. These clients need to be heard and validated. For some, healing can begin if their parents apologize.

Other common themes experienced by DCP whose conception stories were withheld from them until adulthood are:

- Feelings such as anger, confusion, relief, curiosity, and sadness.[10]

- Lack of parental support and/or a feeling of guilt/betrayal from parents when wanting to learn more about their own biological identities, ancestry, and more about their close genetic relatives.

- Searching for a deeper understanding of forgiveness which can be an integrative process with conflicting feelings.

Keeping conception stories secret from children can, and often does, cause lifelong harm. This story shared by a donor-conceived person illustrates some of the ways this happens:

When I was an early teen, I had this fantasy that I had a secret identity, which would eventually be revealed to me later. I've never admitted this to anyone until now. It wasn't a grandiose secret identity — just mysterious and a total wildcard that would eventually make sense. I had no idea why this idea cropped up at the time because who I was and where I came from seemed so obvious. (I wasn't told about my conception.) But how appropriate that was, in hindsight.... I had real problems with my sense of identity until about 2 years ago (when my truth finally and shockingly emerged through technology) and had been inhibited in the public eye because of it. Asperger or introversion or family dynamics or just plain uniqueness were once the theories for this tendency, but there was obviously something else going on that made me feel like the odd woman out and made me want to retreat. There are so many things I've wanted to do but could never complete due to shaky confidence in who I was and what I had to offer. (For example, singing.)

This problem has been melting away quickly of late, and things are very clear now, like a light has been switched on. Secrets are felt viscerally, even when they aren't explicitly known, which is why they can be so toxic. And to fully build out who you are, you need to know where you came from. It's easy for those who don't know what this is like to take what they had for granted and tell you to get over it, because 'all that matters is who you choose to become.' But there's a primal need in all of us to understand our roots first (at the parental level) — before that can happen — like a psychological foundation for individuation. I've had an incredibly fortunate and privileged life and loving parents, for which I've always been grateful, so this isn't me bellyaching in a spoiled way. It's just that some things can't be replaced by a nice lifestyle or all the love in the world. Humans are weird, with all our specific needs. Wish it could be simpler.

DCP who have already had many years, or a lifetime, to incorporate their conception stories into their overall identities may be less likely to present for treatment for this particular issue. These people may be neutral, accepting, and even embrace their donor origins and may even incorporate their new donor family into their existing family with ease, regardless of when or how the information was disclosed.

Even if these individuals are presenting for treatment for other reasons, however, it is relevant for the therapist to understand their family systems as they may be referenced in the course of treatment.

In the donor family context, secrecy can imply shame among other factors. Many parents who were initially dealing with the shame and grief of infertility, and the loss of their dream of the perfect family where their children were genetically related to both parents, haven't yet worked through these feelings and emotions. Keeping donor conception as a secret can create a fault line in the family's foundation, and can damage the parent-child relationship without the child ever knowing why, and they can blame themselves.

When DCP in heterosexual families find out the truth, their parents sometimes insist that they too keep the secret, or won't speak about it. In these situations, unfortunately the shame of infertility is passed along to the DCP and manifests as shame of donor conception. Parents who feel inadequate or insecure about their parenting (or themselves) are more likely to pass along these sentiments. These parents are not providing the support that their children need to process through their emotions and feelings. This can make it much more difficult for the DCP to not only accept and process the circumstances of their conception, but also to forgive their parents and mend those relationships, allow themselves to be curious, and to consider searching for and connecting with their unknown genetic family.

DCP finding out later in life are more likely to feel like their identities have been altered and their lives disrupted. For many, psychological work and plenty of time for healing is needed so they can put the pieces back together to reshape their identities and stories. This has sometimes been described by DCP as "genealogical (or genetic) bewilderment", a term coined in the 1950s[11] to describe the identity crisis that adoptees were going through when separated from genetic family and raised with non-genetic family.

Grief, relief, forgiveness

According to available research, around one third of DCP have sought professional support or counseling regarding their donor conception origins.[12-14] Many of those who sought help have learned the truth about their origins later in life, and may therefore be moving through stages of grief that can resemble those of Kubler-Ross's model.[16] For many there are multiple layers of discovery and grief to work through as they process their new truth, learn about what they have lost, and learn they have been lied to for years.[1]

- **Shock**: A rush of strong emotions in response to this unexpected truth is common, as are feelings of instability. *My world has been turned upside down. I am rattled to my core.* This type of shock can feel traumatic if the DCP feels that they can't cope with the stress of learning the truth, or if they can't accept their emotions, or integrate the new information into their personal story. Dismissing or ignoring the emotional impact of learning the truth about their origins instead of figuring out how to incorporate it into their reality can run the risk of buried emotions surfacing later.

- **Denial:** *This can't be. My mother must have had an affair. The DNA company made a mistake. I look just like my mom/dad. My parents would never have lied to me. My parents couldn't have known.*

- **Anger/Frustration:** *Why didn't you tell me? Who else knew? Why can't I know who my close genetic relatives are, or my ancestry, or my family medical history? How many and who are* *my half-siblings? Who is my biological mother/father?* Feelings of betrayal are common in these scenarios.

- **Sadness/Depression**: *I'm sad to know my parents lied, sad to know I am not related to my mom/dad or their family, grieving for the identity I had that will now need to be adjusted. I'm also sad that I can't know my close genetic relatives, ancestry, or medical history.* [5,6]

- **Reconciliation**: Forgiveness. Acceptance. Coming to terms with all their emotions. Searching for answers, and accepting that there might not be enough of them. Feeling comfortable enough to consider reaching out to new relatives to learn more about them and define new donor family relationships.

Contrasting Kubler-Ross's linear model,[16] Pauline Boss offers six nonsequential guidelines meant to help people bear their grief that can also be very helpful when assisting DCP who are feeling loss:

- Make meaning out of loss.

- Relinquishing one's desire to control an uncontrollable situation.

- Recreate identity after loss.

- Become accustomed to ambivalent feelings.

- Redefine one's relationship with whatever or whomever they've lost and finding new hope.

Two of these guidelines, "meaning" and "new hope," are especially important for coping. They are intended to help people consider what the loss signifies in their lives and how they can imagine a future that contains their loss, potential gains, or new family structure.[17]

Loss that is experienced without sufficient resolution, sometimes called unresolved grief or ambiguous loss, can leave a person searching for answers and can complicate and/or delay the grieving process when those answers aren't easily or quickly found. Many DCP experience ambiguous loss after finding out the truth about their conception at an older age, have parents who are not forthcoming with information, can't find sufficient information about their unknown genetic relatives, or when their parents are no longer available to offer the missing pieces of their origin story. If DCP are curious, but can find no answers, they can alternate between hope and hopelessness, but ultimately need to accept that they might not ever get the answers or closure they so desperately desire.

Disenfranchised grief is described by grief researcher Ken Doka as, *"Grief that persons experience when they incur a loss that is not or cannot be openly acknowledged, socially sanctioned or publicly mourned."*[18] DCP feeling a sense of loss from being cut off from their biological family can have their grief ignored, minimized, negated, criticized, misunderstood, and dismissed by others who might not understand or accept this type of loss for a family never known. They might have a disrupted schema, with a need to restructure the way they view themselves in relation to others and the world, including giving up their prior vision of themselves and their family. It's not uncommon for DCP to have their pain dismissed with the "you should just be happy to be alive" argument. Yes, DCP are usually very happy to be alive, but that doesn't preclude their feelings of discontent. Some DCP are hesitant to express their feelings of grief within their families or friend circles because they fear they will be labeled as "ungrateful". It's important that DCP feel safe, validated, accepted, and supported in their grieving process. Counselors can provide guidance and interventions for disenfranchised grievers as they navigate through the social interactions that may include unhelpful expectations and judgments.

It's also possible that the DCP hasn't been able to adequately express their grief (or other emotions) because of difficulty with processing and verbalizing their related feelings. They might also feel confused about who they can talk to and have fears of over-sharing with friends, co-workers, or acquaintances. They may struggle with telling their parents (or siblings they've grown up with) that they now know the truth about their conception for fear of upsetting them and rocking the family's foundation. It's important for the client to not feel as though they need to keep this information and experience as a secret. Connecting with other DCP on the Donor Sibling Registry or via other support groups is one way that their feelings and emotions can be normalized and supported.

It is not uncommon for some DCP to report feeling relieved when they finally learn the truth, as many suspected *something*[7] because of so many differences between them and their family, overhead conversations, or non-verbal clues in the family. Many have reported thinking that their mother had an affair or that they were adopted. Many feel that they have been manipulated as their suspicions and inquiries were dismissed and denied. The clear message was that they then couldn't trust their own instincts. For these people, learning the truth includes recognizing that they weren't "crazy" to suspect that they were not related to one or both of their parents or that they had a biological family in addition to the one they grew up with.

Forgiveness is a crucial step in a DCP's healing process. Feelings of hurt, shame, sadness, or confusion can be lying underneath the more visible emotion of anger. Because empathy is a significant component of forgiveness, DCP can be encouraged to process their emotions by better understanding the context or story of their parents while holding them accountable, and at the same time remaining in touch with their humanity. Forgiveness can be similar to grief work as it's processing disappointment and deciding how to best move forward. Your client may also need to hear permission to be in a place of unforgiving, with understanding and validation that the process is being worked on. Parents' apologies for not telling can go a long way in facilitating and accelerating a DCP's forgiveness process.

DCP have a wide range of curiosity levels. Sometimes the level of curiosity is based upon the family type that the person comes from.[2] For example, do they have a positive family experience? If not, maybe the thought of inviting more people into their close family circle might not be comfortable. Do they have underlying mental health struggles like depression or anxiety? Do they have family support? Do they have a non-biological parent? They might feel a sense of betrayal to their non-biological parent if they reveal any curiosity about their potential or newly known genetic relatives. A DCP might not have the emotional bandwidth to explore new family relationships. It can be scary to open yourself up to possible rejection or to weave (many!) new family members into existing family fabrics. This can be true for both healthy and less intact families.

Many DCP are excited to learn that they are donor-conceived and look forward to connecting with their new expanded family. Some are happy to know that they cannot inherit some of the mental or physical illnesses from their non-biological parent. Some are thrilled to begin the adventure of making their new familial connections. When DCP have their parents and other close relatives and friends walking beside them, the journey is more satisfying and easier, especially if there are challenges along the way.

Attachment styles

Attachment style can indicate how open or fearful DCP are when exploring, initiating, creating, or maintaining relationships with new genetic relatives.[19] A secure attachment style may allow for easier processing of feelings and emotions when considering making new connections and moving forward to establishing new relationships. Anxious, dismissive, or fearful attachment styles may make it more difficult to even consider reaching out or responding to new genetic relatives or following through with exploring the nature and possibilities of these new relationships.

A 2016 study of donor-conceived adolescents found that those who were securely attached were more willing to engage in the sometimes challenging task of exploring donor conception, those who demonstrated evidence of insecure attachment were more likely to show a preference for avoiding the topic of donor conception altogether, and those who demonstrated insecure dismissive attachment were least likely to express curiosity at all.[20]

Another study of 447 DCP adults in 2018 examined whether individual differences in attachment relate to self-reported curiosity about one's donor conception and a person's choice to find or contact their donor. Interestingly, results indicated that participants high in attachment anxiety were more curious about their donor conception, albeit disengaged from it, and that insecure attachment, particularly attachment anxiety, may contribute to a person's willingness to incorporate donor conception into his or her identity but not necessarily to act on it. The study also found that DCP who were anxiously attached to their parents were more likely to exhibit curiosity about donor conception, potentially as a means of offsetting their unmet attachment needs. This suggests that greater attachment anxiety might lead individuals to exhibit curiosity about their DCP identities. In doing so, they may seek out communicating with other DCP or acquire further information about donor conception as a way of managing their anxiety.[21]

Curiously not curious

Sometimes, DCP insist that they are not at all curious about or interested in meeting their half-siblings or their other biological parent. Although this is true for some, this ambiguity or outright disinterest is sometimes rooted in:

- Feeling ashamed or embarrassed about the way that they were conceived, and not wanting to acknowledge or think about it.

- A feeling that any curiosity they might have will be perceived as a betrayal of sorts to the parents who are raising them, particularly to the non-biological parent, even if their parent(s) are deceased.

- Thinking that their parent(s) would disapprove of any curiosity and/or a desire to meet, or that parents would be disappointed or hurt in some way, especially if parents have minimized/negated/dismissed the importance or significance of the child's unknown biological parent or family (sometimes, parents give a clear message, both action and inaction can speak louder than words, that the donor or half-siblings would not be a welcomed addition to their lives or into the family circle).

- Concern that the sibling(s) they've grown up with or other family members won't approve or will be hurt.

- Fear of rejection and/or fear of not being good enough, or not having accomplished enough, or not being mentally stable enough, or just not being at the "right place" in life.

- Fear of learning that the biological parent who contributed 50% of their DNA will be flawed in some way, which might then impact their own sense of personal identity.

- Fear that meeting genetic relatives will somehow take away from their current family relationships, family system, and family stability.

- Worry that they'll be disappointed with their new relatives or that they won't have enough in common.

- Concern about not having the emotional bandwidth to deal with a meeting, or with incorporating new relatives into their lives, especially if there are many of them.

- Worry that friends, family, or others will be judgmental — e.g., *"Those people are not your family."*

DNA Matters: psychological issues

Many studies on DCP have shown that a primary reason for searching for one's biological parent and/or half-siblings is the importance of learning more about their family medical history, current medical issues, and possible pre-dispositions. A 2021 survey asked 529 DCP for the main reason that they wanted to be in touch with the donor. While 26% said, "to feel complete as a person", a close second, 23%, wanted to learn more about their medical history.[12-14]

Although most people acknowledge the heritability of many physical attributes and diseases, the correlation between genetics and psychological illnesses, disorders, abilities, and traits is less understood. Robert Plomin, who has studied twins and adoptees for fifty years, explains in his book, *Blueprint: How DNA Makes Us Who*

We Are, that genetics accounts for 50% of psychological differences, not just for mental health and school achievement, but for all psychological traits, from personality to mental abilities.[22] DNA isn't the only factor, but it is the most significant in terms of the stable psychological traits that make us who we are. He believes that all psychological traits are heritable, about 50% on average. Plomin's foundational 1985 research also concluded that genetics is generally responsible for about half the correlation between parenting and children's psychological development.[22,23]

So, while the parents that raise and love us contribute to who we are, our DNA blueprint holds an immense amount of information about both our physical and mental selves. Genetic research results tell us that schizophrenia is up to 50% heritable, autism is at 70%, reading disability 60%, and even personality scores 40%.[24] Knowing one's close genetic relatives can be helpful, and even crucial for DCP to better understand their psychological selves.

Questions and topics to explore with the DCP client

As scientific study of thoughts and feelings common to the DCP is ongoing, typical questions and topics that frequently arise continue to be identified.[1,2,15,25-28] In terms of current knowledge, here are some additional topics that may be discussed further in therapy sessions:

- How does the client define "family" and how do they view both nature and nurture as contributors to who we are?

- Does the client understand that new donor connections have the potential to enrich all of their lives?

- How important to the client is learning about one's ancestry?

- How important is it to learn about one's close genetic relatives, e.g. grandparents, and half-siblings?[25]

- The importance of learning about one's family medical history.[27]

- Does the client want the donor to know they exist and that they are someone to be proud of?

- Will the client respect the boundaries of the donor and other DNA relatives?

- The possibility of learning that their mother's doctor is actually their biological father.

- The possibility of learning about a sperm bank mix up such that the gametes their parent(s) purchased (along with the donor profile) is not their actual biological donor parent, or that the sperm bank or donor lied on the donor profile, and they could end up learning that there is no information about which donor their parents used.

- Discovering that their biological parent (or half-sibling) is not someone they would normally interact with, and addressing differences in socio-economic status, political, religious, or other core belief structures.

- Learning that the sibling they grew up with is really a half-sibling.

- Finding out about mental or physical illness with their newly found half-siblings or with their biological parent/donor.

As these topics are explored, it is relevant and important to know that desired connections with the donor are not money-driven (i.e., that the donor should pay for education), DCP are not "looking for a dad," and DCP do not desire to invade/disrupt the lives of donors or half-siblings. It's an innate human desire to know where and who we come from, about our ancestry, and about our family medical history.

Recommendations for adult DCP who just found out

Encourage your client to talk with their parents and other supportive family members and friends. Many people have walked this path before, and although the road can get a bit bumpy for a little while, they have all survived. Secrecy implies shame, and your client has nothing to be ashamed of, so do not let the "secret" persist.

- **Ask questions.** Encourage your client to ask their parents why they used a donor and what the experience was like for them. Ask why they kept the secret. Most parents don't tell because they were advised not to by the doctors and/or they're afraid of how the truth will affect their families. Often, the non-biological parent is afraid of being seen as not the "real" parent or having their status as a parent somehow diminished. Your client can assure his or her non-biological mom or dad that this news does not have to change the parent-child relationship. The more emotionally honest everyone involved is, the easier it will be for the DCP.

- Encourage your client to explain very honestly how this news has affected them, and help them understand that their feelings about their conception story may change over time. For many DCP, finally learning the truth may for the first time allow them to know that they can trust their own instincts. Difficult feelings are normal to have in this context; this was their information to have, and it was kept from them. It can be very important to acknowledge what parents can't yet say or apologize for. Working through these feelings may take time. For those who found out on their own, or were told as adults, it is important for them to know that they are owed an apology from their parents for not being told the truth sooner.

- **Listen.** Your client's parents may have made the best decisions they could with the information they had at the time. Many parents were advised to lie to everyone, including their children. In the subsequent decades, many were too afraid to acknowledge that this truth was something that children deserve and the lie that was damaging to the family system and relationships. Some parents were lied to about "sperm mixing" and believed that the donor's sperm was mixed with the father's sperm to make the father's sperm more "potent". Couples were also told to go home and have sex after the procedure, obfuscating the fact that a donor was used and almost certainly would be the biological father. Encourage your client to find out what their parents know about the donor or any half-siblings. Gathering information about the other half of their genetic identity and relatives may help DCP better understand themselves. Many offspring report feeling a sense of relief as they reassemble the puzzle of their physical, emotional, and intellectual selves.

- **Forgiveness is essential.** Your client may never fully understand or agree with their parent's reasons for keeping this information from them. Working through the anger is necessary for forgiveness to occur. Clearly communicating with their parents about the need to hear words of apology and acknowledgement is crucial for the rebuilding trust process. Empathy and compassion will be extremely helpful in repairing any damaged relationships. It's important for DCP to understand that forgiveness may be the only path to true healing and acceptance. It's important for parents to know that they can be forgiven for not telling the truth, even if this might take some time.

- **Continue the conversation.** This is not a one-time conversation. Encourage your client to let their parents know that they will ask them to continue the conversation as they process this new information, tell family and friends, and incorporate it into their identity. Encourage your client to invite their parents to walk beside them as they explore their genetic roots and learn what it means to be a DCP. There is great opportunity for a stronger family bond if your clients can keep the lines of communication open as the family will now be grounded in truth. Your client can invite their parents to love and support them in this journey.

Your client needs to accept their new reality and understand that any curiosities they have about half-siblings and/or their unknown biological parent, ancestry, and medical history are normal and to be expected. Your client can't change the past, but they can control how they move forward. This is their story to own and share as they see fit.

If your client is curious and does desire to know more about their donor family, you can give them resources so that they can search for the information and the genetic relatives they're curious about. Their curiosity is not a betrayal to their parents, particularly to the non-biological parent, in any way. Adding new family members or ancestral information doesn't take away from or diminish the importance of the family that loved and raised them. Work with your client so that they can manage the feelings and emotions that arise when little or no information is found right away. It can take time for answers to come, so patience is required. The same is true for when their genetic relatives are found, and the path forward isn't so easy or so clear.

A note on clients conceived via embryo donation

Although embryo donation is a newer form of assisted reproductive technology, and although most conceived through this method have not yet reached adulthood, there is a great likelihood of individuals conceived in this way presenting for therapy in the future. Research has yet to focus on this topic, however, it can be projected that similar thoughts, feelings, and courses of action from the DCP group will extend to this group. Embryo-conceived people will be similar to adopted people in that they won't have much information about 100% of their genetic, ancestry, or medical backgrounds. Further complexities may occur as embryo-conceived individuals may have different sets of siblings from the maternal, paternal, and joint sides of the family.

Now that you have gathered the initial information about your client and their experience of being a donor-conceived person, just as with any client presenting with a new area of focus it is important to educate yourself on the topic. Reading this guide is a great start.

> *If we know where we came from, we may better know where to go. If we know who we came from, we may better understand who we are.*
> ~Anonymous

My feelings are difficult to explain to people who take their roots for granted. An adopted person once described the sensation of what is now termed 'genealogical bewilderment' as having to drive through life without a road map. I find it to be an apt description of my situation. People who know both of their biological parents find it hard to grasp the enormity of what I am missing. Simply having information about the sort of people they are, and what things they are capable of doing, creates a baseline that you don't realize is comforting unless you have to live without it. **-DCP**

I feel that my perspective of feeling blessed to be a donor-conceived person, thus to be who I am, isn't typically portrayed as strongly or as often as the perspective that there is a void or sadness attached to being conceived from donor insemination. I think the main reason that I am so comfortable with who I am and how I was conceived comes from the honest and loving way in which my mother approached the topic with me, at a very young age (the very first time I asked why our family was different than my friends' families). She explained my conception as a blessing that was only possible because she wanted to have me so badly and because a wonderful stranger donated half of the ingredients she needed to make me who I am.

Of course there is curiosity about what I don't know, but it doesn't ever negatively affect me. If I someday learn more, it would just be a blessing on top of all of the blessings I've already had in my life. I love my life, I love who I am, and I love everyone who has contributed to that. **-DCP**

I am a donor child. My mom didn't tell me till I was 21. I always knew something was different; I used to constantly ask if I was adopted. I never felt a sense of belonging. However, I wish my mom would have told me sooner. The way she went about telling me wasn't the best situation either and everyone always knew, it was a secret that was kept from only me. I am now almost 26 and a recent parent myself. I find myself wanting to know more and more about who my "dad" is, even if it is just medical history, etc. as when I became pregnant with my son, there were so many questions asked about medical history on each side of the family and I couldn't answer them. I think if my mom would have told me sooner I might be more comfortable with the situation. It is rough not knowing who your "dad" is. **-DCP**

References

[1] Bertisch, H. & Kramer, W. (2021). The donor conceived adult: Implications within family, medical and mental healthcare systems. *Advance Medical and Clinical Research*, 2, 16-17.

[2] Jadva, V., Freeman, T., Kramer, W. & Golombok, S. (2010). Experiences of offspring searching for and contacting their donor siblings and donor. *Reproductive Biomedicine Online*, 20, 523-532. doi:10.1016/j. Rbmo.2010.01.001

[3] van den Akker, O. B., A., Crawshaw, M. A., Blyth, E. D. & Frith, L. J. (2015). Expectations and experiences of gamete donors and donor-conceived adults searching for genetic relatives using DNA linking through a voluntary register. *Human Reproduction*, 30, 111-21. doi: 10.1093/humrep/deu289

[4] Blyth, E., Crawshaw, M., Frith, L. & Jones, C. (2012). Donor-conceived people's views and experiences of their genetic origins: a critical analysis of the research evidence. *Journal of Law and Medicine*, 19, 769-89.

[5] Canzi, E., Accordini, M. & Facchin, F. (2019). 'Is blood thicker than water?' Donor conceived offspring's subjective experiences of the donor: a systematic narrative review. *Reproductive Biomedicine Online*, 38, 797-807. doi: 10.1016/j.rbmo.2018.11.033.

[6] Macmillan, C. M., Allan, S., Johnstone, M. & Stokes. M. A. (2021). The motivations of donor-conceived adults for seeking information about, and contact with, sperm donors. *Reproductive Biomedicine Online*, 43, 149-158. doi: 10.1016/j.rbmo.2021.04.005.

[7] Beeson, D., Kramer, W. & Jennings, P. K. (2011). Offspring searching for their sperm donors: how family type shapes the process. *Human Reproduction*, 26, 2415–2424. https://doi.org/10.1093/humrep/der202

[8] Scheib, J. E., McCormick, E., Benward, J. & Ruby, A. (2020). Finding people like me: contact among young adults who share an open-identity sperm donor. *Human Reproduction Open,* Volume 2020, Issue 4, 2020, hoaa057, https://doi.org/10.1093/hropen/hoaa057

[9] Indekeu, A., Bolt, S. H., Janneke, A. & Maas, B. M. (2021). Meeting multiple same-donor offspring: psychosocial challenges. *Human Fertility* (Cambridge), 12, 1-16. doi: 10.1080/14647273.2021.1872804. Online ahead of print.

[10] Jadva , V., Freeman, T., Kramer, W. & Golombok, S. (2009). The experiences of adolescents and adults conceived by sperm donation: comparisons by age of disclosure and family type. *Human Reproduction*, 24, 1909-19. doi: 10.1093/humrep/dep110

[11] Sants, H. J. (1964). Genealogical bewilderment in children with substitute parents. *British Journal of Medical Psychology*, 37, 133.

[12] Siegel, D. R., Sheeder, J., Kramer, W. & Roeca, C. (2021) How experience frames donor-conceived people's feelings about utilizing donor-assisted reproduction themselves: insights from individuals conceived via donor-assisted reproduction. Abstract published in *Fertility and Sterility*, 116, 3 supplement E433. doi: 10.1016/j.fertnstert.2021.07.1159E433

[13] Siegel, D. R., Sheeder, J., Kramer, W. & Roeca (2021). The age and by whom a donor-conceived person receives information significantly affects their experience. Abstract published in *Fertility and Sterility*, 116, E431-432 supplement. doi: 10.1016/j.fertnstert.2021.07.1156

[14] Rushing, J., Siegel, D. R., Kramer, W., Sheeder, J. & Roeca, C. (2021) Do donor-conceived people become donors themselves? Abstract published in *Fertility and Sterility*, 116, 3436 supplement. doi: 10.1016/j.fertnstert.2021.07.1166

[15] Hertz, R, Nelson, M. K. & Kramer, W. (2013). Donor conceived offspring conceive of the donor: The relevance of age, awareness, and family form. *Social Science & Medicine*, 86, 52-65.

[16] Kubler-Ross, E. & Kessler, D. (2005). *On grief and grieving: finding the meaning of grief through the five stages of loss*. New York, Scribner.

[17] Bernhard, M (2021). What if There's No Such Thing as Closure? Many of us are taught that if we work hard enough we'll be able to get over our losses. The social scientist Pauline Boss sees it differently. *New York Times*. https://www.nytimes.com/2021/12/15/magazine/grieving-loss-closure.html?campaign_id=52&emc=edit_ma_20211217&instance_id=48076&nl=the-new-york-times-magazine&regi_id=68745685&segment_id=77269&te=1&user_id=d88ff65750cb81847362276fdd3b8fe0]

[18] Doka, K. J. (1989). Disenfranchised grief. In K. J. Doka (Ed.), *Disenfranchised grief: Recognizing hidden sorrow* (pp. 3–11). Lexington Books/D. C. Heath and Com.

[19] Flaherty, S. C. & Sadler, L. S. (2010). A review of attachment theory in the context of adolescent parenting. *Journal of Pediatric Healthcare*, 25, 114-21. doi: 10.1016/j.pedhc.2010.02.005

[20] Slutsky, J., Jadva, V., Freeman, T., Persaud, S., Steele, M., Steele, H., Kramer, W. & Golombok, S. (2016). Integrating donor conception into identity development: adolescents in fatherless families. *Fertility and Sterility*, 106, 202-208. doi: 10.1016/j.fertnstert.2016.02.033

[21] Lozano, E., Fraley, R. C., & Kramer, W. (2019). Attachment in donor-conceived adults: Curiosity, search, and contact. *Personal Relationships*, 26, 1-14 doi:10.1111/pere.12273

[22] Daniels, D. & Plomin, R., (1985). *Differential experience of siblings in the same family*. *Developmental Psychology*, 21, 747–760.

[23] Oliver, B. R., Trzaskowski, M. & Plomin, R. (2014). Genetics of parenting: The power of the dark side. *Developmental Psychology*, 50, 1233-1240. doi: 10.1037/a0035388

[24] Knopik, V. S., Neiderhiser, J. M., DeFries, J. C. & Plomin, R. (2017). *Behavioral Genetics*, 7th Edition. Worth Publishers, New York, NY.

[25] Persaud, S., Freeman, T., Jadva, V., Slutsky, J., Kramer, W., Steel, M., Steele, H. & Golombok, S. (2016). Adolescents conceived through donor insemination in mother-headed families: A qualitative study of motivations and experiences of contacting and meeting same donor offspring. *Children & Society*, 31, 13-22, doi: 10.1111/chso.12158

[26] Hertz, R., Nelson, M. K. & Kramer, W. (2017). Donor sibling networks as a vehicle for expanding kinship: A replication and extension. *Journal of Family Issues*, 38, 248–284, doi: 10.1177/0192513X16631018

[27] Crawshaw, M., Daniels, Bourne, K., Adams, D., Van Hoof, J. A. P., Pasch, L, Kramer, W. & Thorn, P. (2015). Emerging models for facilitating contact between people genetically related through donor conception: a preliminary analysis and discussion. *Reproductive Biomedicine & Society*, 1, 71-80. doi: 10.1016/j.rbms. 2015.10.001

[28] Nelson, M. K., Hertz, R. & Kramer, W. (2013). Making sense of donors and donor siblings: A comparison of the perceptions of donor conceived offspring in lesbian-parent and heterosexual-parent families. In: *Visions of the 21st Century Family: Transforming Structures and Identities Contemporary Perspectives in Family Research*, Volume 7. Emerald Group Publishing Limited.

[29] Adams, D. H., Gerace, A., Davies, M. J. & de Lacey, S. (2021). Self-reported mental health status of donor sperm-conceived adults. Journal of Developmental Origins of Health and Disease, 31, 1-11. doi: 10.1017/S2040174421000210. Online ahead of print.

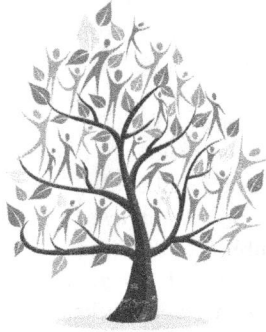

CHAPTER 5

Parents of Donor-Conceived People

Exploration of the thoughts and feelings of the biological and the non-biological parents

It is important to understand the themes that commonly arise with parents of DCP. Given the historical secrecy surrounding donor conception, there was little empirical literature in the area until the last few decades, and this area of study continues to evolve.

Both available research and numerous anecdotal accounts do suggest themes in the experience of the parents of donor-conceived people.[1]

- Grief/sadness/shame over infertility and/or pregnancy loss and how that can affect their child. Unresolved infertility grief is all too often passed along to the child as shame in the form of secrecy. Ideally, healing work in this area would be done before a DCP is born.

- Loss of hope for their own or their partner's genetic connection with a child. Sadness or fear over what that means for their future family.

- Privacy/secrecy issues and the desire to hide the use of a donor. Keeping such a big secret from everyone is a lot of work and can be exhausting.

- For SMCs, the shame of not having a partner. Sometimes, parents use the desire for "privacy" to mask the unrealized embarrassment of not having a partner.

- For those who conceived when they were single, and then married when their kids were older, there might be worries about how to incorporate their new spouse into the existing family system.

- Struggling with choosing the right donor. Curiosity or fear about their child's donor: what they look like, potential medical issues, or what kind of person they are. Will they be ok carrying the baby of a stranger?

- Financial concerns. Have they saved enough money for a maternity leave and do they have good insurance that will cover costs should any medical complications arise as a result of their pregnancy, the birth or in their newborn?

- Worry that other children will tease their DCP because of the difference in their family.

- Worry about how accurate the donor or the gamete vendor was with the information they were given about the donor. Most gamete brokers now provide a medical sheet that is a snapshot of one day in the life of a healthy young donor, with medical updates rarely asked for or accepted and shared with families. Sperm can be sold for decades.

- The desire to protect themselves or their child behind the (false) screen of anonymity.

- Disclosure: trying to decide if, how, and when to tell their child and others about their use of a donor. Fear about the child's reaction to the news especially if the child is older. Possible discord in a marriage if one parent wants to tell, and the other doesn't. It can be important for parents with adult children who haven't yet been told to hear words of acceptance, empathy, and forgiveness, all while encouraging them to tell.

- Discomfort when their children want to talk about their unknown genetic relatives.

- Potential contact worries: will their family be negatively affected by making contact with their child's half-sibling families or donor? Will the donor be receptive?

- What if the child ends up liking/loving the donor more than them?

- The legal and emotional issues that might present themselves if using a known donor, (a friend, family member, or stranger found via social media).

- Changing definition and experience of "family."

LGBTQ+ parents

Research published by the Family Equality Council provides some insight into how many lesbian, gay, bisexual, transgender, and queer (LGBTQ+) people are interested in becoming parents, and how they are planning to do so. Most significantly, the data reveal dramatic differences in expectations around family building between LGBTQ+ Millennials and older generations of LGBTQ+ people.[2]

Key findings include:

- 63% of LGBTQ+ Millennials (aged 18-35) are considering expanding their families, either becoming parents for the first time, or by having more children.

- 48% of LGBTQ+ Millennials are actively planning to grow their families, compared to 55% of non-LGBTQ+ Millennials, a gap that has narrowed significantly in comparison to older generations.

- 63% of LGBTQ+ people planning families expect to use assisted reproductive technology, foster care, or adoption to become parents, a significant shift away from older generations of LGBTQ+ parents for whom the majority of children were conceived through intercourse.

In the early decades of donor insemination, many clinics, doctors, and facilities did not allow LGBTQ+ people (or single women) to purchase donor sperm, but now approximately a third of parents buying sperm are LGBTQ+ couples and singles.[1] These parents of donor children are not dissimilar to heterosexual parents, in that many also raise their kids in emotionally rich and stable environments. Children in LGBTQ+ families are often acquainted early on with the knowledge and belief in tolerance and diversity. LGBTQ+ families can, however, have unique stresses including in healthcare, schools, and with legal parentage issues. The non-biological LGBTQ+ parent is not always properly acknowledged and can face discrimination or feel like they are being dismissed.

Counselors can convey ease, acceptance, inclusive language, terminology and pronouns (non-binary language is always evolving), and provide LGBTQ+ people with inclusive and welcoming words, materials, websites, intake forms, and policies.

The non-biological parent

Many people who are considering having a child face the possibility/probability of not being genetically related to that child. Whether they're a man, woman, or couple dealing with infertility or a genetic issue that makes it impossible to have a biological child, or they're an LGBTQ+ couple, and they choose to use donor eggs or sperm, someone in their family equation will be in the position of being the non-biological parent.[3]

Many non-biological parents have not been adequately counseled or educated before using donor conception to create their families. It is vital that these parents deal with any loss, grief or shame that they may have around their own infertility, work through any emotions they might be experiencing from the lack of biological connection, and educate themselves about the needs and issues their child might have before a child is born. If a non-biological parent has unresolved emotional issues, they could accidentally signal their discomfort, pain and/or shame to the child, which can cause the child to feel shame in being donor-conceived.

Unfortunately, many parents still try to withhold the truth from their children to protect the non-biological parent. Family secrets can be toxic, and we believe that these parents, expecting honesty from their children, *owe their children the same.* In families with secrets, all too often the "secret" hovers just beneath the surface, creating distance between non-biological parents and their donor children. The DCP can be unsure why there is a feeling of distance between them and their non-biological parent. This disconnect can have life-long negative consequences.

Parents who do disclose the truth can still pass along their insecurities and fears with regards to their child having any type of curiosity about, and wishing to connect with their unknown biological family. It is often the non-biological parent that feels more insecure about their parentage, and the child can be affected by this insecurity.[3] Never speaking about it again, or giving the child the clear message that it's an uncomfortable subject and not welcome to be discussed can have significant circumstances for the child and for the whole family dynamic. Not making peace with their lack of biological connection may create discourse and guilt within the child when any natural feelings of curiosity arise within them.

These issues can arise for both heterosexual and LGBTQ+ families. We hear all too often that the non-biological mom in an LGBTQ+ family, for example, may minimize the contribution of the donor, which could be harmful to a donor-conceived child trying to construct their identity and acknowledge all contributors. Sometimes the non-biological parent is afraid of a child reaching out to half-siblings and/or their donor, and says things like "biology doesn't make a family." These parents' unresolved discomfort or sadness about not having a genetic connection to their child can cause great instability and insecurity within their nuclear family. Often this is expressed as disappointment or anger at a curious child, causing the child to then feel a great sense of betrayal even just thinking about the unknown people they are genetically related to. This can be paralyzing to the DCP who have a longing or desire to explore connections with their unknown relatives and actually make efforts to do so.

Sometimes a DCP learns or figures out the truth, but they still shoulder the secret. Research and anecdotal information give evidence that quite often, adult donor offspring have found out that they were donor-conceived, but we're afraid to tell their non-biological parents that they knew for fear of hurting them. In this case, the secret becomes intergenerational, as the children themselves are also struggling to keep the "secret" that the parents have also shouldered for so long. These DCP people frequently feel acutely aware that the methodology of their conception causes pain to their non-biological parent, and therefore willingly accept the weight of this pain to carry themselves. This only enforces the idea that the way they were created is somehow shameful and should be kept secret.

In the beginning, parents make all the choices about how their child will come into the world. These are choices that will affect children for their entire lives. But it isn't only about what makes parents most comfortable. They must also ask, *"What is in the best interests of this child to be born?"* Reading research and testimonials from donor-conceived people is strongly suggested before making any decisions. What may be just a "donated cell" or a "piece of genetic material" to a parent, often means a lot more to a DCP. Parents need to be very careful not to put their own fears and biases onto their children and allow them to process for themselves the meaning of "family" as they mature. DCP are brought into the world using a methodology that disconnects them from one-half of their genetic background and relatives. It's important to honor and respect any desires they have to seek out this unknown or "invisible" family, and parents can offer to walk by their children's side as they explore and make their donor family connections. Doing so leads to stronger family connections.

In our published research of 244 non-biological parents, there was a difference between non-biological mothers and fathers over whether they were interested in meeting their child's other biological parent, the donor. 73% of the women who utilized donor eggs indicated that they would like to meet the donor while only 45% of the men (who utilized donor sperm) indicated interest.[4] Adequate counseling and education and working through one's own grief and fear as well as understanding their children's desire to know about their ancestry, medical background, and roots before pregnancy would save a lot of donor families from heartache. Making peace with the concept of not being genetically related to their children is essential for non-biological parents to create an honest, respectful, and healthy family with strong bonds. Exploring what it means to be a parent and acknowledging that their children are a wonderful blend of both nature and nurture can lead to peaceful and loving relationships. Yes, DCP are deeply influenced by the parents that love and raise them and also by the parents that contribute 50% of their DNA. Understanding and respecting this fact, and that knowing where and who one comes from is an essential ingredient in the formation of a donor-conceived child's current and future identity is vital for having a healthy family.

Telling

Shouldering the secret and the associated guilt can be a heavy burden for parents to carry. Just like families with adopted children, the secret can create needless negative implications. There are so many reasons to disclose the truth to family, friends, and most importantly, to the donor-conceived children.

Disclosure is a common theme seen in those seeking the services of helping professionals. It is best to talk with children about their origins from when they are preverbal. That way, parents can practice talking about the issue in a positive and affirming manner and children can then easily incorporate the information into their identity with no traumatic "telling" event. Children love hearing the story of their origins, and there is no time too early to begin unfolding their story.

When we talk about telling, we are talking about being open and honest, particularly with the donor-conceived child about the use of donor gametes. Children can understand very basic concepts at an early age about the sperm, egg, and the difference between the parents that raise, love, and take care of them and the biological parent that gave the sperm or egg to help create them, but that they might not ever get to meet. Telling also includes the parents modeling disclosure conversations to friends, family, teachers, doctors, etc. so that the child learns how to not only better understand, but also how to explain their origin story to others. A parent's comfortable and accepting tone is just as important as the content of the information they're relaying. This is especially relevant when and if the donor becomes known, and how the donor is then positioned by the parents within the family context.[3] There are children's books that explain donor conception in a simple and gentle way. One book that also addresses half-siblings and donors is *"Your Family: A Donor Kid's Story."*[6]

When a DCP finds out by accident or later in life about their conception, there is often trauma, distress, anger, or confusion. In a survey of 741 donor-conceived people, the age respondents learned of the method of their conception had a bearing on whether they felt confused upon learning this new information. Of those who said they had "always known", 9% indicated that they felt confused about their conception, while 46% of those who had not been told until they were over 18 felt confused.[5]

What are the reasons that parents give for not telling?

- It wasn't important. They saw no reason to tell. This is sometimes cover for deeper unresolved issues.

- They "forgot about it". This is very unlikely and also may be used to avoid discussing other unresolved issues.

- They claim to not have known that the doctor had used donor sperm, also unlikely.

- They believed the idea of sperm mixing. In the 1940s-1980s heterosexual couples facing male infertility were often told that the doctor would mix the husband's sperm with the donor's to make the husband's sperm "stronger". This fallacy allowed the couple to have hope that the husband was indeed the biological father. Couples were also told to go home and have sex after the insemination, obfuscating the truth of the donor being the biological father of the resulting child.

- Fear that the truth will be too heavy a burden, or just too painful for their child. This is particularly true for parents who struggle to accept the use of a donor themselves.

- Too afraid to tell as the child might be upset or very angry with them. *If I don't talk about it, I can avoid pain, for my child and for me.*

- They think their child is too young or not yet mature enough. This excuse can be used indefinitely to avoid disclosure.

- Religious or cultural reasons for parents feeling that they must keep donor conception a secret.

- Too busy and never the right time: kids in school, kids preparing for finals, kids' mental health issues or medical issues, moving, changing schools, divorce, other trauma in the family, etc.

- The other parent doesn't want to tell and they don't want to create discord in the relationship.

- Fear of the non-biological parent being viewed as "less than" by the child and/or others (friends, family, acquaintances, strangers). In reality, DCP often report that the relationship with their non-biological parent is stronger after disclosure, as it then becomes a relationship grounded in honesty. In families created with donor sperm, it is common for the adult DCP who just found out to initially place more anger on their biological mom as more complicated feelings, including empathy, are more focused on the dad.

- Fear that the stable or unstable family system might implode when the truth comes out.

- Afraid of their child not being able to find out any information on their donor family.

- Fears that connecting with the newly-found genetic family will take away from the existing family, or negatively affect the current family structure.

Recommendations for parents of a DCP: telling early on

- Encourage clients to talk with their children openly and early about their stories. Donor-conceived children need to have the details of their conception story be part of open and ongoing discussions to keep shame and conflict out of the equation. When children are little, telling can be as simple as a bedtime story about how they were born, becoming more detailed as they grow and mature. *Your Family: A Donor Kid's Story*[6] is a children's book that can assist parents in introducing and discussing the concepts of egg/sperm/embryo donation, different types of families, curiosity, and half-siblings and donors to young children.

- Your clients will be ready to answer new questions from their donor-conceived children, and able to continue the conversation. By the time children start elementary school, there will be visits with friends, and assignments in school, such as family trees, that will bring the conversation to the forefront. Beware the mistake of assuming that children don't want to talk about their families and how they were conceived if they don't ask. Children are usually curious. If parents don't make their conception stories an ongoing conversation, their children may think it is a taboo subject, or hurtful to their parent(s), or they might also interpret that the way they were conceived is something shameful.

- Encourage clients to be open about their children's conception stories with the key people in their lives. Knowing helps teachers understand if donor-conceived children say something about it in class, and can help them prepare a way to make children comfortable when the conversation or art projects turn to Mother's or Father's Day. Doctors must know so they are aware that the non-biological parents' medical history has no relevance to the child. Conducting role-plays in session may help the parent practice how to present this information and answer questions so that they become more comfortable doing so.

- When parents of DCP model open, honest, and matter-of-fact conversations about donor conception for their child, they not only set the tone for the context of these conversations in the future, they also demonstrate for their children how to talk about it, thus equipping them with the conversation skills they will need in the future. Families and relationships are topics everyone encounters as they move through life. Preparing DCP for these conversations is as essential for their well-being as is preparing them for school, for driving, and for eventually living on their own.

- Encourage clients to be prepared for their children's potential curiosity and desire to search for their half-siblings and/or their biological parents. They should consider the probability that their children have half-siblings, and how affirming it might be for them to be connected to others with whom they share close genetic ties.

- Clients must also be prepared for their children not finding enough information about their donor relatives. It can take months or years to make a connection, and sometimes connections are not found. This can be frustrating and sad for DCP. It is important to honor these feelings and emotions.

- Encourage clients to view new donor family connections as adding to their families, not taking away from it. Getting to know new relatives does not replace the people that raise, love, and care for their children. It simply means that their children may have more people in their lives who love them. Many parents of DCP embrace their child's donor family and feel reassured that their child will have others for love and support when they are no longer around. Plus, they may find new friendships among people with similar life experiences.

- Sometimes donor-conceived children may have emotional, cognitive, or developmental difficulties that impact the way they process information. In such cases, it may be helpful to start conversations with older children about donor conception in the context of a session with a therapist or counselor whom the child already trusts. Such professionals can then continue to help them understand their story for as long as needed. Ideally, these therapists should have knowledge of donor conception.

Tips for parents of donor-conceived adults who are about to tell or who have DCP who have found out on their own

- **When is the best time to tell? Now.** This is not a parent's secret to carry. There will never be a "perfect" time, so the sooner, the better. It's important that parents do the psychological work necessary to be emotionally capable to have the conversation and adequately support their children, including talking about and understanding the reasons why they haven't told before now.

- **Remind them that this process can be very positive,** affirming, and lead to a more honest and open family system with relationships now based in truth.

- **Parents can tell their stories and how they decided to use donor conception.** Remind these parents that they are setting the tone for all future conversations about their children's conception, and should try to keep the conversation light, using some humor if possible. They need to be as grounded, calm, and as level-headed as possible, because their donor-conceived children will look to them for answers about why their conceptions stories were kept from them. Openness and honesty are crucial.

- **Explain very honestly why they haven't told before now.** Parents shouldn't be defensive or use their personal stories as an excuse. Donor-conceived people want and deserve to hear the truth and the *emotion* behind why they were not told earlier. What were they or their spouse afraid of? Knowing all of this can help their children adequately process through their own emotions, which might include anger, sadness, confusion, or even relief, while also feeling empathy towards their parents.

- **Parents can let their children know that they made the best decisions they could with the information they had at the time.** Many parents were advised by their gamete vendor or doctor to keep the secret. They can tell their children how it has felt to carry this information as a secret and how they've recently come to learn about the importance of honesty. Parents should also tell their children who else knows.

- **Share any and all information.** For parents with children born before the 1980s (fresh sperm), they may have little, if any, information about the donor, while most parents with children born from the 1980s through present time (frozen sperm) usually do have a donor profile or some other non-identifying information about the donor that can be shared.

- **Most important: Apologize. Own it.** In both scenarios where DCP learned the truth on their own, or when parents disclose it to them as adults, it's important for parents to apologize. This was their children's information to know, and the parents kept it from them for too long. Parents can empathize and keep apologizing as necessary to allow their children to move freely through their emotions without getting stuck in anger. Sometimes, DCP want their parents to feel the hurt that they do as they feel as though the parents are responsible for it. Parents with adult children who need more time to process their emotions or who may resist letting go of their anger can be supported to stay the course, and be reminded to take care of their own emotional and physical selves during this time. The road ahead might be a bit challenging for a while.

- **Recognize the negative implications of asking children to keep the "secret".** Secrecy can imply shame and/or guilt. DCP can respond negatively when asked to carry on the shame of infertility in the form of secrecy. This is a burden that should not be passed along from parent to child.

- **Parents should be ready to continue the conversation.** This is not a one-time conversation between parents and their donor-conceived children. Some parents make the mistake of telling, but then never talking about it again. This gives their children the idea that the topic of their conception story is unwelcomed or too shameful to discuss. It's very important that DCP know that their origin stories are a welcomed, ongoing conversation and that they will be there for them as they process this new information, tell family and friends, and incorporate it into their identity. It's ok for parents to disclose their own discomfort while admitting that they too are on a healing journey. Parents can gently broach the topic regularly if their children don't, so that the DCP knows they're there to help them understand what this new information means to them and their life.

- **Telling is just the first step.** Parents must make sure their adult children know that any curiosities they have about their half-siblings and/or their unknown biological parents, their ancestries, and their medical histories are normal and to be expected. If a parent is not fully comfortable with this, it's important they understand why, so they can continue to grow and heal in this area.

- **If their children are curious…** If their children desire to know more about their origins, parents can offer to walk side-by-side with them to find the information and genetic relatives they want to know about. Parents should understand that their children's curiosity is not a betrayal in any way. If they are uncomfortable helping their children learn more, they can honestly express that in a way that lets their children know their discomfort is not their fault, and that the parent is actively working on it. This is especially important for the non-biological parent. Parents can be reminded that how they feel today may be very different from how they'll feel in 3, 6, or 9 months from now and that they, and their families, can continue to evolve together around these issues.

- **It's important for DCP to know that many others have walked this path before them.** Parents can share that while their child's conception story may seem unique, their origin story is certainly not uncommon and there are opportunities to connect with other DCP via the Donor Sibling Registry and on various other social media groups. Parents of younger adults should be alerted that there are some DCP social media groups where excessive anger is the norm and therefore might not be appropriate for DCP still trying to put the pieces together in a healthy, empathetic, forgiving, accepting, and positive way.

Not every case of a DCP finding out about their donor conception later in life results in trauma. Sometimes, if parents are open, honest and patient, the telling can result in a meaningful conversation that opens the door for more. From a young donor-conceived person:

I am 13 years old and in 8th grade. My name is Lauren and I am also a twin. I found out about a month ago now that my dad wasn't my real biological dad. I was shocked at first but then the next day I was excited to tell my friends the news and curious about the donor and what he looked like. I know that my dad is my real dad and will always be, but I still wanted to do some research about the donor. That night I sat on the couch with my family and we all went through the packet about the donor (heritage, looks, health, etc.)

Now that you have gathered the initial information about your client and their experience of being a parent to a DCP, just as with any client presenting with a new area of focus it is important to educate yourself on the topic. Reading this guide is a great start.

> *There are only two lasting bequests we can hope to give our children.*
> *One is roots; the other wings.*
> ~ Hodding Carter

Watching the pain/struggle that I know my 19 year-old son feels with wanting to know the donor breaks my heart. I say in hindsight that I think the child has rights; the right to know the other parent. Rights that I as the mom ignored or underestimated at the time I made the decision to have him.- **Parent**

I would imagine the question that some of you will ask is "Was his world "rocked?" after my son learned the details of his conception. I can honestly answer that at this moment in time, he has embraced this unique side of himself with amazing poise, grace, and at times, humor. He has accepted his fate and seems to have found a new sense of who he is. It's not that he was unhappy with himself before, but this new sense of identity finally meshed with the one he was living with inside. It was always difficult for him to understand why he was so different from his Dad both in personality and physicality, and this new information just brought more balance into his life and an understanding of why he felt so different. I have read so many stories from donor-conceived children who felt that they had sensed something was different all of their lives, and I believe in his own way, our son also sensed that things weren't as they were being portrayed. **-Parent**

My husband and I had always intended for him to know eventually. We just never knew when that time would come. For me, every child deserves to know who they are and where they came from. Do we as parents have the right to keep that from them? To quote a donor conceived child, "It was like looking into a mirror and seeing only half of my reflection" after he found out how he was conceived. Our child deserved to see his entire being every time he looked into a mirror which made the search for his donor that much more urgent. I also am of the opinion that the more people in the bleachers cheering for your child to succeed in life, the better. As parents, we are not perfect, and if we had the means to put just one more individual in his life, such as his biological father, to help guide him through the murky waters that lie ahead, then we owed him that. In our case, he didn't just gain one individual, but an entirely new set of family whom I believe will be cheering for his well-being from here on in. What a gift to give to a child. **-Parent**

One common problem that we've seen in the lesbian community (and to a lesser extent in the gay community) is the idea that if you talk about the donor, you are implicating the family in being somehow less than enough and implying that two women or two men alone do not make a family.

This is a reaction to a very serious political situation. Yes, there are also attacks on women who have children without fathers — but single female parents are also not denied any fundamental rights. They are not constantly being told that they are not a family or that one of the parents does not matter. There is no danger that their child will be taken away from them or that they would ever be denied custody.

In this context of sustained attacks, a common reaction is to assert that the family is perfect and there is no need to talk about the donor. Gay people are often very defensive about their families and thus reluctant to talk about the donor. Many people have said that they refuse to talk about the donor to anyone because they perceive doing so to be questioning the legitimacy of their family — so they refuse to engage in that conversation. Families should not be built based on fear and defensiveness. We owe more than that to our children. -LGBTQ Parent

References

[1] Sawyer, N., Blyth, E. Kramer, W. & Frith, L. (2013). A survey of 1700 women who formed their families using donor spermatozoa. *Reproductive Biomedicine Online*, 27, 436-447, doi: 10.1016/j.rbmo.2013.07.009

[2] Family Equality: LGBTQ Family Building Survey. https://www.familyequality.org/fbs (December 17, 2021).

[3] Widbom, A., Isaksson, S., Sydsjö, G., Svanberg, A. S. & Lampic, C. (2021). Positioning the donor in a new landscape-mothers' and fathers' experiences as their adult children obtained information about the identity-release sperm donor. *Human Reproduction*, 38, 2181-2188. doi: 10.1093/humrep/deab146.

[4] Frith, L., Sawyer, N. & Kramer, W. (2012). Forming a family with sperm donation: a survey of 244 non-biological parents. *Reproductive Biomedicine Online*, 24, 709-18. doi: 10.1016/j.rbmo.2012.01.013

[5] Beeson, D., Kramer, W. & Jennings, P. K. (2011). Offspring searching for their sperm donors: how family type shapes the process. *Human Reproduction*, 26, Pages 2415–2424, https://doi.org/10.1093/humrep/der202

[6] Kramer, W. & Moore, J. (2018). *Your Family: A Donor Kid's Story*. Donor Sibling Registry, Colorado.

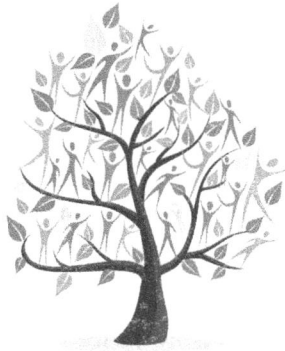

CHAPTER 6

The Sperm or Egg Donor (the Biological Parent of DCP)

Exploration of the thoughts and feelings of the donors

Themes that all clients considering selling their gametes should consider

If your client is thinking about selling their gametes, it is important for them to consider the ongoing ramifications for themselves, their families, and for any children born who will share approximately 50% of their DNA. If your client sold their sperm or eggs very recently, their genetic material may be sold for many years, or even decades into the future. Some things to consider:

- **Medical Issues:** Specifically for women thinking of selling their eggs: there are unknown medical risks resulting from egg donation, and few longitudinal studies to date. Depending on the length of time since treatment, donors have reported coping with unpleasant short-term side effects such as changes in menstrual cycle, ovarian hyperstimulation syndrome, an immune reaction, or muscle/joint pain. Some have also had to cope with more long-term issues regarding their own (premature) infertility following IVF, concerns about decreased ovarian reserve, or breast cancer due to potential long-term effects of hormonal stimulation, which have not been well-researched to date.[1,2] Former donors have reported feeling angry that they had not been well-informed about the possible medical risks of egg donation, as many clinics indicate that there are "no known risks" of egg donation, because there have not been sufficient long term studies.[2]

- Should your client (who is considering selling their sperm or eggs) or a member of their immediate biological family develop a medical or psychological issue following the initial completion of the self-reported medical history on the donor profile, it would be crucial to share this information with the families who purchased their gametes. It's not just their looks, intellect, or athletic abilities that might get passed along. Susceptibility to disease is also often inherited. Often diseases don't develop until later in life, so for many years after the original donation, children who share their DNA may develop medical and health concerns that sometimes can only be properly addressed with updated information. Conversely, it might be important for your client to know about any medical issues reported by their extended families, as they may affect their own current or future children. Certain conditions carry genetic components that are not readily tested for, and accurate information is vital for proper screenings, testing, and preventative care.

- **If your client has children of their own or plans to....**Has your client considered the possibility that in this small world their children may encounter biological half-siblings? At the present time, gamete vendors do not keep, nor are they required to keep, any record of live births resulting from any specific donor. What this means for the children born with their DNA (whether donated or not) is that there may be many half-siblings. The children a potential donor has now, or may have in the future, may someday meet their half-siblings, the biological children born from their donations. Random meetings among half-siblings have historically occurred, so honesty is essential. Before they donate, potential donors should consider their willingness to be forthright with their spouse/partner and children. There are ramifications of these potential meetings beyond mere curiosity. Consider the potential problems that could occur from a romantic relationship with a half-sibling.

- **"Anonymous" donations...**It is important to understand that because of advances in DNA testing and Internet search engines, the likelihood of your client remaining anonymous in the future is unlikely no matter what they are told by a gamete vendor. Even if your client does not do DNA testing, their progeny would match with any member of their family who does and can then trace the path back to your client. It is important that the client consider the likelihood that they will be contacted by progeny or their parents. How would they respond if they were asked to meet with their genetic offspring?

- **The future.** Have they considered how they might feel about their donations in the future? It is likely that more than one child will come to exist as a result of their donations. These children are genetically the client's offspring; in fact, they may one day have children of their own who will be your client's genetic grandchildren. If they haven't yet told their family about the donations, they will need to think about the fact that this could be potentially disruptive to any family that they may have formed in the traditional manner. If they have been open with their family, and their spouse/partner/children/parents are open to meetings, this can be a time of excitement about the possibility of expanding family.

- **Imagine how their donor offspring might feel.** Many will wonder about where they got some of their physical characteristics. Or wonder about who they get their talents, mental abilities, and personality traits from. Many are extremely curious about genetic family history and ancestry, and many feel a deep longing to connect with and to know their unknown genetic parent.

- **Imagine their reaction if their genetic offspring found them and expressed a strong desire to connect, or if they needed life-saving medical treatment.** Your client needs to consider these issues carefully as they make their decision on whether or not to sell their gametes. Their actions today may have an incalculable effect on the future.

- **The client needs to understand that their donation is much more than a business transaction with a gamete vendor.** They are, in most cases, helping to create new lives. This truth can reverberate across a donor's life.

One egg donor reflects on her donation experience:

Infertility. This word never really stuck to me until I started my journey of being an egg donor. I am blessed to be healthy, but deep down, I knew there was something more I could do. This is when I decided to look into egg donating. I have since then been matched twice on DSR. One of the recipients of my eggs is someone I have met and communicate almost daily with. It took communicating with one of my recipients to truly see the impact I have made in the life of this couple. I really started seeing the bigger picture. These eggs are the answers to many - many prayers of some people. "Positive pregnancy - give me a baby."

I am very thankful that I have been able to play such an important role to the couples who received my eggs. I hope to hear from them if they decide to educate their children about how they were conceived. I am grateful that these recipients chose me to hold such an important role in their lives. It is so rewarding to me to know that I have helped so many people in the short time that I have been on this Earth.

My relationship with one of my recipients is very strong. We communicate daily. The relationship I have with this couple is a bond I never even thought I could have. It isn't the typical relationship you have with a friend - cousin - wife - husband. It is an unexplainable bond and relationship that only someone else who has donated or received eggs from a donor would understand. My appreciation and respect go out to my recipients. I welcome anyone to reach out with any questions, as I am sure there will be many.

Common thoughts and feelings surrounding the experience of being a current or former gamete donor

It is important to understand the themes that commonly arise with this population. Both available research and decades of anecdotal reporting suggest themes in the experience of current and former sperm and egg donors that you may expect to be reported in the context of assessment and treatment sessions. These include:

- Reasons for donating include financial gain (egg donors may make up to $10,000 or more for a single donation, while sperm donors can make more than $16,000 in the minimum one year donation contract), helping families who wanted children, enabling other parents to enjoy parenting as they have[3] or to "pass along my genes."[4]

- There may be frustration about a lack of pre-donation education or counseling and feel that they were not prepared for the possibility of contact with any resulting children born as a result of their donation under a false concept of anonymity.

- Curiosity about offspring.[5,6] Many wonder if their offspring think of them, have concerns about the wellbeing of children created, and feel frustrated about not being able to know or contact them.[4] One study suggests that about three-quarters of donors have feelings about wanting to contact donor children and not being able to; another quarter feels worried about their donor children's well-being.[3] Although older research suggested that few egg donors had actually made contact,[3] new research tells us that a majority of egg donors would like to make contact with offspring, and now have the means to do so as thousands of donors have made mutual consent contact on the Donor Sibling Registry and via other methods. Ninety-four percent of surveyed sperm donors were open to contact with offspring, with 85% being open to meeting them and 78% open to establishing a relationship with them.[7]

- Concerns around anonymity. Many donors donated long before commercial DNA testing existed, and more recent donors were not provided with information about DNA companies like 23andme and Ancestry.com that could be used in the future by children from the donation to contact them. Younger donors may be more neutral as many were given a choice of whether to be anonymous for 18 years or forever. Older ones may be more biased towards wanting to meet offspring.[3] The ones who favor anonymity may want to protect the parents from feeling threatened or want to protect their own families or their own lying by omission about being a donor and/or having medical issues. Many have fears about their relatives being contacted via the DNA websites.

- Once the realization that contact is not only possible but probable, there can be fears about their parental rights and responsibilities, including financial responsibilities or liabilities (there are none), or a fear of rejection or not being liked or accepted.

- Fear or embarrassment associated with their family and friends finding out that they sold their gametes and/or that there are resulting children. It is common for donors to sell their gametes to more than one, or many, facilities. These donors may worry about being exposed for their serial donating history.

- There may be thoughts and concerns about the numbers of offspring that have been created using their donated gametes. Most egg donors feel that it is important/very important to know the number of offspring born from their donations.[3] Some clinics try to provide this information, although more than 40% of surveyed egg donor parents say that they were not asked by their clinic to report the birth of their child.[2,8] Although earlier research suggests that sperm donors have generally been neutral on limiting the number of offspring by clinics,[6,9] with the increasingly widespread use of the Donor Sibling Registry and of DNA testing, many now understand that they were lied to about the limits of the 10 or 20 offspring that they were promised.

- Many sperm donors feel overwhelmed by the implications of how many offspring they have, as some have come to find out that they have more than 100 or even 200 donor children. There may be concerns over how large numbers of offspring might demand too much of their time and/or attention and therefore affect their family negatively.

- Fears about disappointing the offspring or not being successful or good enough. Some donors were not 100% honest about their academic backgrounds when filling out their donor profiles and now feel ashamed.

- Feelings of rejection as many DCP with non-biological parents see connecting with the donor as a betrayal of sorts, and therefore do not wish to establish relationships. DCP who are worried for and protecting their non-biological parents can appear as though they are rejecting the donor.

- Feelings of guilt after finding out about medical issues amongst their donor offspring that they could be responsible for, or shame if the medical issue was something they hid in order to be accepted as a donor.

- When a donor attempts to report updated medical information or history that may affect their current or potential offspring, there may be frustration over the dismissive responses and lack of follow-up from their gamete vendor, and the lack of guidelines for how to provide this information.[6]

- Many donors are excited to learn about and connect with their donor progeny and now reports of donors connecting with their donor-grandchildren are becoming more common.[6] Many need some time and patience to figure out how to define these new relationships with their genetic children and their families. Creating new family systems can be a bit of a challenge as the process unfolds until relationships become better defined and accepted.

Specific to egg donors:

- Former egg donors have reported anxiety and depression which may make them likely candidates for psychotherapy.[7]

- Earlier research suggests that about half of egg donors feel that their relationship with their offspring is only genetic, while the other half view it as a connection beyond biological.[3] More recent 2021 research asked egg donors how they viewed any children who may have resulted from their donations. The most common response was "special designation but not acquaintance, friend, or family"(36%), and the second most common was "my biological child" at 26%.[7]

- Fears about how the egg retrieval process might affect their future health and fertility.

Questions and topics to explore with donor clients

As the scientific study of thoughts and feelings common to individuals who have sold their gametes is ongoing, typical questions and topics that frequently arise continue to be identified. In terms of current knowledge, here are some topics that may be discussed further in therapy sessions:

- How do they feel about having been a donor? Themes may include pride, shame, embarrassment, fear, excitement, and ambivalence. Have these feelings changed over time?

- How do they feel about the anonymity?

- Do they think about their donor children or worry about their happiness and well-being?

- How comfortable are they regarding to sharing information about having donated with parents, close relatives, friends, children, and more distant people (i.e., co-workers, on social media) in their life.[3]

- Have they searched for their DNA offspring or have donor children found them?

- Are they worried about balancing their current families with their newly found donor children? Do they have support from their spouse/partner?

- Have they rejected contact from their donor progeny? Do they feel as though that's a door that will never be opened, or is their possibility for a change of heart?

- Do they feel as though they were properly counseled or educated about the potential curiosities of their donor children? 80% of 164 surveyed sperm donors and 66% of 109 surveyed egg donors said that they did not feel like they were adequately counseled about the potential curiosities of the children that would be born from their donations.[2,4]

- How do they feel about not being given the opportunity to share updated medical and genetic information through the gamete vendor, despite the desire to act responsibly?[4]

- Do they wonder whether and how to connect with donor children? Thousands of egg and sperm donors have made themselves available for mutual consent contact via the Donor Sibling Registry. Earlier studies suggest that donors are open to contact with offspring but the methods vary.[4,6,10] This has likely changed with the increased use of DNA testing resulting in connections with older offspring, many of whom did not know the methodology of their conception.

- Have they been rejected by donor offspring or their families? Some donors have reached out but not received replies or ongoing communication from offspring or their parents. In many instances this is not because of who the donor is, but rather an indication of other factors with the offspring and their families. Sometimes the explanation is as simple as a change of email address that was not updated in the Donor Sibling Registry.

- Are they concerned about a large number of donor children? Finding the time and energy to connect or establish relationships with many donor children can seem overwhelming. How might they gradually unfold this process with perhaps one or two families at a time?

- If they are considering contact, are they worried about rejecting or hurting donor children due to not being able to meet their expectations? How can they balance building relationships with offspring with not feeling like they are intruding on their lives or being perceived as a threat to their parents?[6] Exploring how to set healthy boundaries with offspring and families is an important step.[4]

Telling family and friends about donor history

Egg donors are likely to have told others in their lives, including their partners, friends, and siblings about their donation and they are somewhat likely to have told their parents and their own children.[3] The majority of surveyed sperm donors were also likely to have shared about their donations with their wives and children.[4] For those who haven't yet told, telling others may come to the forefront as they consider contact or after an offspring has made contact with them.

Although some research suggests that donors feel that their offspring should not be kept secret from their own families,[4,6] many may be embarrassed, afraid, and/or unsure of how to tell them, and it may still be a secret. In other cases, families may know and be supportive.[4,6] The best way to tell is to simply be straightforward and open to answering questions. Many parents of donors are thrilled to learn about and make connections with their donor-grandchildren.

After contact has been made, some donors may view offspring as part of their extended family and almost half come to feel the same way about the parents of their donor offspring.[6] However, there can be adjustment within the donor's family once actual contact is made with donor offspring.[4] For a donor with their own family, it may be helpful to think of two families engaging or merging with each other, rather than thinking about one big donor family."[4]

Donors understanding why DCP desire contact: What's it all about?

It *is* about:

- Learning about ancestry.

- Learning about family medical history.

- Learning about other close genetic relatives, such as grandparents and the donor's other children, their half-siblings.

- Wanting the donor to acknowledge that they exist – acknowledgement.

- Wanting the donor to know that they are someone they can be proud of – recognition.

- Wanting to give the donor the opportunity to know them.

- Wanting the donor to know that they will respect all boundaries.

- Wanting the donor to understand that this connection could enrich everyone's lives.

It *is not* about:

- Money, e.g., paying for education.

- Looking for a dad or a mom, or someone to actively "parent" them.

- Invading or disrupting the donor's family or life in any way.

Here's an example of "what it is all about" from a DCP who shared this story:

They felt like family, and for me there was a sense of relief in that too. Like it's hard to put a finger on it but I think a good analogy would be like finding people who speak the same dialect as you. Like I've been trying to speak [my last name] all these years and it just never came naturally to me and it was always a struggle and I didn't know why. Then I found out it's because I was speaking [donor's last name] the whole time and discovered that talking to my half-siblings and biological father is so much easier and intuitive in a way I haven't experienced before.

Mutual consent contact and the Donor Sibling Registry

The Donor Sibling Registry is a way for donors and their offspring (through the offspring's legal parent for minor children) to make mutually desired contact. Unlike connections through DNA testing, when donors register on the DSR, they can remain private if wished, and they'll know that connection is desired on both sides. Many egg donors have connected on the DSR right from pregnancy or birth of the child, as many egg facilities write this into their parent-donor agreements. This methodology may be more difficult for older DCP without a donor number or much donor information to go on. Please see Chapter 7, *Connecting: Donors, Parents, and DCP* for more information.

Now that you have gathered the initial information about your client and their experience of having been an egg or sperm donor, just as with any client presenting with a new area of focus it is important to educate yourself on the topic. Reading this guide is a great start.

While I have been quite at peace with the decisions I made years ago, the stories of these children pull strongly at my heart. I feel bad now that I really never considered what the opinion was of the children involved, and possibly selfishly, though unintentionally, deprived them of something that they may need at a level I never understood or considered. **-Sperm Donor**

Having been an egg donor, I think every day about any and all of the children I have helped create for other families. I think about what stage of childhood they are at, and just curiosity about who they are, and will someday become. I also think about all the parents I have been blessed to help with my gift. **-Egg Donor**

I want all my genetic offspring to be happy and healthy like my own children. I will always love them and wonder where they are, what they are doing, if they are living, learning, and experiencing life like me and my own children. I hope that they are bringing the same joy to the lives of all the mothers and dads the same way my life has been enriched by my own children. We are, and will always be, connected. Some of them will become equally as curious as I was some day, and want to know more. I think we owe it to them to let them learn. I think there are many reasons a donor father might want to get involved with a genetic offspring. I think though that those reasons change over time as we grow older and wiser. **-Sperm Donor**

It's not just donor-conceived people who are genetically linked to each other by their donors. It's also the extended families of the donors- their wives, parents, children who are part of that family tree. My children have half-siblings out there somewhere because my husband donated sperm as a college student with an iron-clad anonymity contract. My children had no say, any more than the children who were born via that donation had any say in it, but that doesn't make them any less genetically related.

I don't feel threatened by the fact that there are potential children out there my husband fathered through this decision he made years ago. It is what it is. I believe my children have the right to know if there are half-siblings out there that resulted from their dad's donation. If all parties are willing to know one another, why not let them? It doesn't take anything away from me as a mother or, I don't think, from the parents of donor-conceived children. Families will remain intact, the circle of knowledge will only grow and more of the puzzle pieces fit together for all of these children (and adults). **-Wife of Donor**

Many years ago, when I was a lot younger and at university I found a poster on campus talking about egg donation. At the time I didn't think twice about it, I just knew deep down that there are wonderful people out there who have so much love and affection and compassion to give but for one reason or another God has not given them the opportunity to have a baby. It saddened me, why there are people who live a callous existence and are able to have children but these amazing people aren't. The world truly seemed unfair to me even then. I made my decision there and then to be a help and not a hindrance in whatever way I could to people wanting to be a parent. But that was one side of the picture. Over the years, some of the people I had donated to wanted to stay in touch with me and at the time I refused. I didn't want to complicate their lives nor my own. Now I am older and with children of my own, I realize what it was they are asking of me. Looking back at all I had experienced and the letters I had shared with recipients, that connection is special. I understand now why they would like to stay in touch and I am open to it now. -Egg Donor

References

[1] Schneider, J., Lahl, J. & Kramer, W. (2017). Long-term breast cancer risk following ovarian stimulation in young egg donors: a call for follow-up, research, and informed consent. *Reproductive Healthcare*, 34, 480-485, http://dx.doi.org/10.1016/j.rbmo.2017.02.003 1472-6483

[2] Kramer, W., Schneider, J. & Schultz, N. (2009). US oocyte donors: a retrospective study of medical and psychosocial issues, *Human Reproduction*, 24, 3144–3149, https://doi.org/10.1093/humrep/dep309

[3] Jadva, V. Freeman, T., Kramer, W. & Golombok, S. (2011). Sperm and oocyte donors' experiences of anonymous donation and subsequent contact with their donor offspring. *Human Reproduction*, 26, 638–645, https://doi.org/10.1093/humrep/deq364

[4] Daniels, K., Kramer, W. & Perez-y-Perez, M. V. (2012). Semen donors who are open to contact with their offspring: issues and implications for them and their families. *Reproductive BioMedicine Online*, 25, 670– 677, doi: https://doi.org/10.1016/j.rbmo.2012.09.009

[5] van den Akker, O. B., A., Crawshaw, M. A., Blyth, E. D. & Frith, L. J. (2015). Expectations and experiences of gamete donors and donor-conceived adults searching for genetic relatives using DNA linking through a voluntary register. *Human Reproduction*, 30, 111-21. doi: 10.1093/humrep/deu289

[6] Hertz, R., Nelson, M. K. & Kramer, W. (2015). Sperm donors describe the experience of contact with their donor-conceived offspring. *Facts, Views, and Vision in Obstetrics and Gynaecology*, 7, 91-100.

[7] Adlam, K., Koenig, M. D., Patil, C., Salih, S., Steffen, A., Kramer, W. & Hershberger, P. E. (2021). The disclosure experiences of egg donors across the lifespan. Poster accepted to the annual conference of the *Midwest Nursing Research Society* (MNRS).

[8] Blyth, E., Kramer, W. & Schneider, J. (2013). Perspectives, experiences, and choices of parents of children conceived following oocyte donation. *Reproductive Biomedicine Online*, 6, 179-88. doi: 10.1016/j.rbmo.2012.10.013

[9] Nelson, M. K., Hertz, R. & Kramer, W. (2016). Gamete donor anonymity and limits on numbers of offspring: the views of three stakeholders. *Journal of Law and the Biosciences*, 3, 39–67, https://doi.org/10.1093/jlb/lsv045

[10] Jadva, V. Freeman, T., Kramer, W. & Golombok, S. (2011).Sperm and oocyte donors' experiences of anonymous donation and subsequent contact with their donor offspring. *Human Reproduction*, 26, 638–645, https://doi.org/10.1093/humrep/deq364

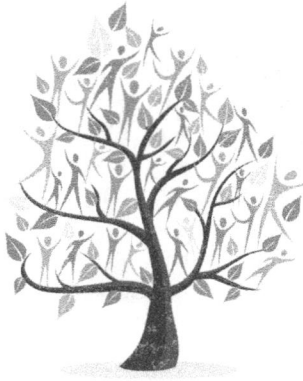

CHAPTER 7

Connecting: Donors, Parents, and DCP

Expanding family

For some, new donor family connections are immediately filled with excitement and enthusiasm, and for others more time to process the information is first needed. In addition to acknowledging their own emotions, some may need to think about how these connections will also affect their family members, including parents, siblings, children, and partners.

Love over fear

- When faced with opening their lives to unknown genetic relatives all donor family members might feel fear, confusion, or worry, and they can make choices solely based on these feelings. There is an opportunity in these situations, to make choices coming instead from a place of love and possibility.

- Parents can put the needs and desires of their children to seek out and connect with half-siblings and/or donors, above their own fears. Allowing their children to grow up knowing their half-siblings can be a wonderful gift they give to their children, and to themselves. Honoring children's right to explore these new half-siblings and/or donor relationships can strengthen bonds within the family.

- Donors can also open their lives to new possibilities of expanding family. All donor family members can choose to see the opportunities in reaching out and connecting, cautiously and carefully, to expand their own or their child's definition of family. Donor's children can greatly benefit by being able to grow up knowing their half-siblings. Donor's parents often are thrilled to know about their biological grandchildren.[5]

- The benefits of exploring donor family connections can largely outweigh any concerns that people might have. These connections have the ability to empower and give people another opportunity to show confidence, love, and support when meeting and embracing newly found family.

As noted above, donor's children can benefit from knowing their half-siblings. For some it can fulfill a deep longing, as in this story shared by the child of an egg donor:

Years ago my mom sold her eggs to help pay rent and give us a good holiday (we weren't doing well at the time). I was around 7 at the time and didn't understand until now how big of a deal that was. I'm 14 now and it keeps me up at night that I have 1 or more siblings out there. I've been reading stories online about how donor siblings found each other and it literally brought tears to my eyes. I want to meet them so bad and it makes me upset thinking I could go my entire life without meeting someone related to me. I wanna know what they're like ... so bad. I can't even describe how much I want to meet them ... it hurts a little. I've talked to my mom about this and she says just leave it alone and don't think about it too much ... but it's hard. She doesn't know I'm looking for them on the DSR, and I don't know if I'll find them, but I wanna try.

Recommendations for parents and DCP exploring contact and building relationships:[1,2]

- There is no evidence or research that supports keeping DCPs, or anyone, from their half-siblings or a biological parent for 18 or more years. By contrast, the field of mental health has always recognized the benefits of people growing up being able to know and establish relationships with their close relatives.

- When parents or DCPs first match with a donor, a half-sibling, or the parent of a half-sibling, they may experience feelings that they were not anticipating when they first registered on the Donor Sibling Registry, a DNA website, or elsewhere, and therefore they may no longer be sure about what to do next. Allow these clients enough time to explore, and to figure out what they are seeking at this point. Are they interested in a simple exchange of information? Are there questions they want to ask? Is the desire to be "known" to the donor or half-siblings? Do they hope to meet in person? Are they open to expanding their family circle?

- It is perfectly normal to feel ambivalent, meaning that they may experience several simultaneous and contradictory feelings. The strong desire to find a half-sibling or donor can exist alongside the equally intense fear of the unknown. The changes this experience can bring about for themselves, their children, their parents, or to the existing family structure can elicit many conflicting feelings.

- After finding and connecting with new genetic family members, these clients may now have the urge to back out. This can be especially true if there is a huge number of half-sibling families. The same holds true for the donor or half-sibling that they connect with. Sometimes hitting the pause button and taking some time to process the information is the best way forward.

- Parents with non-biological spouses/partners might need to have some first-time conversations about boundaries, their child's genetic relatives, and what these connections and potential relationships might mean for their relationship and for their family. Research tells us that there may be a difference between non-biological female and male parents in their attitudes towards meeting donors and possible siblings of their child, with more women than men being interested in such meetings and that same-sex couples are more prepared to facilitate contact and see a role (e.g. friend, mentor, relative) for the donor.[3,4]

No guarantees, frustration, rejection, or worse

- As in any family, there are no guarantees that your client will like or want to establish relationships with their newly found genetic relatives. A genetic connection is not always enough for a solid family relationship and many people have good reason to be hesitant about being vulnerable enough to the idea of expanding family.

- People are more likely to want to get to know and spend time with family members that they can relate to, who are like-minded, and who share similar interests. There shouldn't be any pressure to establish relationships that feel forced and your clients shouldn't feel like they have some sort of obligation to work on creating a relationship that doesn't unfold naturally.

- For anyone in a donor family who is curious and actively searching, the waiting game can feel very frustrating. Although the chances of connecting with some close genetic donor relatives are pretty good, it is possible that it might take a while, or it might not happen at all.

- Your clients should be emotionally prepared for the potential disappointment of not finding relatives, the pain of being rejected by them, or the grief of finding out that a close donor relative has already passed away. These scenarios can all elicit a similar grieving process for the connection that never comes and a dream that's never realized.

- It can be upsetting and frustrating for a DCP to think about reaching out to a donor that has already been contacted by a few, or by many half-siblings, and has expressed the desire to remain private or to not communicate in any way at all with any of their donor children.

- If a grieving client feels disenfranchised, they might withdraw from their grieving process. They might not acknowledge the reality of the loss and its implications, or might not adapt to the feelings of loss in healthy ways. As a result, their grieving process could remain internal and private, and intensify the process, which increases the risk of complicated grief. This disenfranchised grief can stem from themselves, from friends and family, or even from other health professionals.

- Sometimes finding previously unknown donor relatives can present people that we normally wouldn't relate to or welcome into our lives. Reconciling with those complicated feelings can be difficult, but necessary. We choose who to call family, but not always who we have a biological connection with.

Connecting via DNA or social media websites vs. mutual consent contact on the DSR or elsewhere

There are differences in establishing mutual consent contact and connecting on social media or via a DNA site where this might be shocking news to the clients' genetic families.

- Many people who were unaware of their donor origins have done DNA testing for a variety of reasons: family tree curiosity, the DNA kit was a gift, for medical reasons, a passion for genealogy, they suspect there's a secret, they're looking for someone else in particular, etc.

- It's now very common for DNA testing to provide first- and second-degree genetic relatives, and these results are exposing long-held family secrets. These secrets don't just affect one person, but rather, can affect entire families. Parents who thought they'd keep the secret of using a donor are now being confronted by children who now struggle to understand why their parents were not truthful with them.

- Establishing new friendships and familial relationships via DNA, with people who aren't necessarily prepared for this type of new-relative connection, can be a very different experience than making deliberate mutual consent contact on the DSR or elsewhere.

- People who connect via the DSR are fully aware of their origins and most are delighted to connect with each other. On the other hand, connecting via DNA can be so shocking that some people are just not prepared to even reply to messages from their newfound relatives on DNA websites. For those waiting for a reply that never comes, this can be difficult.

- It is now common for close and distant family members of donors to be contacted by DCP or their parents via DNA websites or via social media. This can put relatives in a quandary about how to respond.

- People add postings on the Donor Sibling Registry for a variety of reasons, and the level of desired contact can certainly vary. There are thousands of members longing to establish relationships with their own or their child's half-siblings and donors, and donors hoping to connect with their biological children. Some members only want to connect to share and update medical information. Many land somewhere in between; uncertain as to what type of contact and relationships they're looking to establish, but willing to explore the possibilities.

- Donor's spouses, siblings, and children also join the Donor Sibling Registry to make mutual consent contact with their own or their children's biological relatives, the DCP. Sometimes they join on behalf of their donating relative, sometimes they join because the donor is unwilling or hesitant, and sometimes it's because the donor has passed away.

- Donor-grandparents are quite often interested in reaching out to their biological grandchildren. One research study asked the parents of donors to indicate their emotional response to learning that they had a DC grandchild. Positive feelings predominated; 61% of those answering this question reported that they felt thrilled, 59% felt excited, and 61% indicated that they were curious.[5]

- Although older DCP (who don't have the luxury of knowing their donor number) might find more success searching via the DNA websites, thousands of parents have joined the DSR during (or before) pregnancy or when their children were very young, understanding the importance of including half-siblings, and even the donors, in their family circle right from the start.

Children meeting their half-siblings

DNA Matters. Donor-conceived people have so much to learn about themselves from what they share with their half-siblings, as physical, medical, and psychological issues and abilities are often shared. DCP's half-siblings inherit around 50% of their DNA from the same biological parent, and although sharing DNA isn't the only way to make a family, it is one way that shouldn't be denied. Half-sibling connections can be celebrated as expanding family can be a wonderful and enriching experience.

The relationships that half-siblings form once they are connected may, in many ways, resemble any other sibling relationship. Beyond the point of contact, if/how they form a new relationship and bond is their choice, and some relationships may be more successful than others. For young children raised knowing their half-siblings, there is no need to figure this out. These people are just their family members. Like other relatives, like cousins, the ones they live nearest to, are most like-minded with, and share the most common interests with are the ones they are more likely to spend time with.

Sometimes donor half-siblings and their parents make multiple connections with their donor half-siblings, their parents, and even with their donor. These connections can and do result in warm supportive relationships that last for years. Sometimes, when all the connections are in agreement, they can meet in person, which can be a very exciting and healing experience, especially for children who felt lonely as only-children in nuclear families. One SMC reports that her only-child enjoys texting one of her nearly same-age DNA siblings because the two girls share the same interests and abilities, including a love of writing stories. The two help each other with plot and character development and really enjoy reading each other's works.

Some parents are concerned that a child under 18 might not be mature enough to handle this type of situation and therefore don't tell their children about known half-siblings, wanting to wait until they are "old enough." Some parents delay by waiting for their child to actually ask about half-siblings. We don't wait for our children to be mature enough or to ask about and meet their cousins or grandparents, so why wait for a child to express interest in other close relatives?

Usually, it's the parents who are much more likely to become overwhelmed with how to define it all. When the parents move forward with meetings in an open-minded, steady, joyful, and confident manner, the kids are more likely to view the meetings as positive. When parents interject their own fears or worries, or thoughts that these half-siblings are not legitimate "family", this can throw unnecessary angst into the connections for the kids.

This donor-conceived person explains why keeping them from their half-siblings can rob them of important connections, relationships and experiences:

> *Just imagine being 20 something and finding siblings on your own when DNA testing is even more wildly popular, or they find you. You then develop some kind of relationship. You find that many of these siblings had parents who encouraged these relationships, even from babyhood. You see the pictures, you hear the stories. Disney, camping, birthdays.... A couple of them will be roomies in college, maid of honor in a sibling wedding, etc. To me, this would be crushing. I would feel so cheated, whether or not I had great neighbor pals, awesome cousins, or even siblings from the same home.*

What can your client expect from contact with the other families they meet? [1,2]

- Your clients can count on finding other families who are also experiencing deep feelings, but just as the circumstances surrounding each child's conception are unique, so are the variations in family structure and reactions to the match. Encourage your client to explore their own comfort levels and openness to exploring possible connections.

- Many DCP have LGBTQ+ or single-mother parents. These families are more likely to share the facts of their conception with their children very early on. For some heterosexual families, this may be their first exposure to different kinds of families, adding an extra layer of stress to the anxiety and excitement of making a match. It is okay to be nervous or unsure about the terms or language that the other family uses. However, heterosexual families that are not open to contacting lesbian, gay, or single-parent families, due to religious or other values, may want to think about those biases before reaching out.

- There is a wide range of depth and breadth and speed with which people connect. Some are held back by their fears, trepidations, and/or their insecurities, many of which are unfounded. Others are interested solely in medical information sharing. Your clients should be prepared for all possibilities. While some families desire a limited exchange of photos and email, but not face-to-face contact, other families are hoping to develop an ongoing relationship that will become a friendship or become extended family. It is best to be clear about the level of connection your client is seeking when they make a match, and try to express that early on so that the other family can adjust their expectations accordingly. Understand, too, that expectations often change over time as comfort levels rise and fears dissipate.

- Your clients may be reaching out to non-biological parents who can feel especially nervous or even threatened by the prospect of their child connecting with people that they have a genetic connection with, something that they themselves don't have with their child.

- Sometimes parents who haven't yet told their children want to meet with half-sibling families and request that the secret be kept by the parents and children who do know the truth. This can be a difficult and unhealthy scenario as asking children to withhold this information and shoulder this type of secret can be harmful and confusing. Secrecy can suggest shame, so this is not a healthy message that's sent to the children who are asked to not tell their half-siblings the nature of their relationship.

For many, meeting other donor conception families is the beginning of meaningful relationships that feel "natural" and last for years. From one LGBTQ parent:

We just returned from a weekend gathering of donor siblings where nine of the twenty-three kids we now know about (while we were meeting, two new families posted on the DSR!) attended along with 2 SMCs, 5 lesbian couples, four grandmothers, and a grandad. The kids range in age from 8 months to 4 years. Like others, we formed a private site to share photos, etc., and have been communicating for about two years. Over the course of the past year or so, several small groups of us have met, but I must say that having such a large group was overwhelming in the best way possible.

I never could have imagined how amazing this would be. I was very hesitant to join the DSR at first for all the reasons I am sure everyone else has. However, meeting the others was not only comfortable but incredibly natural ... like we had known each other for years. The kids warmed up to one another and the other adults immediately, and the other parents seemed like old friends. Not to read too much into the genetics of it all, but there was something truly special about the way everyone interacted. I can't imagine what the future might hold, but I am confident that meeting the other donor siblings and their families was the best thing we could have done for our kids. I am grateful we had the opportunity to begin building these relationships while all of them are still so young. Great memories are being created, as is a healthy and dynamic sense of place for our kids.

Another mom explains her thought process about connecting with half-sibling families and the close connections that she and her daughter now have:

I introduced my daughter to her half siblings early—and back then I was anxious about it as I hadn't yet met Wendy Kramer, and for as much as I thought I knew... I still had much to learn. My anxiety led me to writing down a list of pros & cons, which basically amounted to what could possibly go wrong. I found myself writing, "years from now my daughter stumbles upon the DSR, and based on the date of my post recognizes that I knew of these siblings for years but said nothing... she feels cheated & lied to and I'm left having to explain how I stole all those years from her—years she could have known her siblings." It was after writing that out that I knew I had my answer... these children weren't strangers, they were siblings, and who the hell was I to keep them apart? Contact was made in 2010 and soon thereafter we met. Next to having my daughter, meeting her half siblings and their moms was the greatest thing I've ever done, for my daughter and for me. And to my surprise, it wasn't just the kids that formed relationships—every one of us moms love all the kids (it's kind of impossible not to). So my daughter has not just gained siblings, she's gained their moms, who are closer to her than her aunts, and I gained a sisterhood I never even knew I needed. Opening the door doesn't mean it has to remain opened forever... the kids can opt out anytime they want to... but by opening that door I will never have to face my daughter and explain why I kept her from her siblings.

For DCP (and their parents): recommendations for contacting a biological parent (donor) for the first time[1,6,7,9]

Contacting a biological parent (donor) for the first time can be an exciting yet scary experience. Here is some guidance you can share with your client as they go through this process:

- This can be an overwhelming situation for donors who haven't yet been contacted, or who haven't told their families they donated, or who have family members who are against contact. Your clients will want to get their foot in the door as gently as possible.

- Your clients can reassure the donor that they will respect any and all boundaries. It can be very important for the donor to know they're in control of the situation and the depth and breadth of the unfolding relationship.

- Your client can let a donor know that they don't want to disrupt their family in any way, instead, they just want to give them the opportunity to know them. This should be an invitation, not a demand.

- Your clients can let a donor know that they don't want anything from them — not time or money or another parent, just the chance to know more about themselves (or their children). For starters, your client can explain the importance of knowing about their ancestry and medical background.

- Your clients can also let donors know what type of relationship they would be open to. A friendship? A more familial relationship? What possibilities are they open to exploring? Why do they think that a connection could be fulfilling for both of them?

- Encourage your clients to tell donors about themselves or their children. Such an appeal to a donor's heartstrings can be helpful to make themselves or their kids more than just a vague idea, by including information about their interests or achievements.

- Send photos. Again, this appeals to the donor's emotions. Seeing similarities with the children they helped to create can be profound for a donor who wasn't sure about contact.

- For parents: expressing gratitude can be extremely important.

- Know that if a donor doesn't reply or says "no," it isn't because of who your client is, it's more likely because of their family situation, their lack of emotional bandwidth or a lack of understanding about what connecting might mean for them and their family. Their hesitation might also be about their own physical or mental health issues, fear of not being "good enough," or other issues within themselves or their families.

- Patience is crucial. Sometimes a donor needs some time to work things out internally and with their family members. If your clients get no reply, they can try again in a few weeks or months. If a donor says no, your clients can let them know they're always available if they change their mind. Give them space to hopefully work it out and come around. Everyone needs a pause button, including your clients and their donors.

- Encourage your client to keep the focus on themselves or their children, even if they know about other half-siblings. They can consider sharing that news in upcoming correspondence.

For donors: recommendations for contacting DCP (or their parents) for the first time

Although some donors may have preferred to be anonymous, all gametes sold in the US are sold as anonymous, be it for 18 years or forever, so there is no choice about it. Many of these donors would not have chosen this scenario and we have seen thousands of them who are curious about their progeny and who wish to and who do initiate contact. Many people who donated in the past have had a change of heart and now are open to contact. For those donors, and for the ones who haven't given it much thought, the moment that they match with DCP or the parents they may experience feelings they had not anticipated when they first donated or even when they first registered on the Donor Sibling Registry or via a DNA website, and, therefore, they may not be sure about what to do next. Donors who believed that they would remain forever anonymous might feel fearful or upset about being connected to their unknown biological children via a DNA website or via social media and feel confused about how to inform their families, respond to the inquiry, and proceed.

Allow clients enough time to figure out what they are seeking at this point. Do they need to discuss everything with their family? Are they interested in a simple exchange of information? Is the desire to be "known" to the DCP? Do they hope to meet in person? Are they open to exploring more familial relationships?

It is perfectly normal to feel ambivalent. The strong desire to find offspring can exist alongside the equally intense fear of the unknown changes this experience can initiate in themselves and their families. After having hoped that donor offspring would be found, your client may now have a strong urge to back out, and some may indeed pull back once they have made contact. Because there are no limits on how many children any one donor can produce, and many donors donate to more than one facility, donors might be afraid of opening Pandora's Box of a large group of offspring desiring contact. Sperm donors who were promised no more than 10 or 20 offspring, can be completely overwhelmed at the idea of having and connecting with dozens or hundreds of progeny, and with the advent of egg banks, egg donors may soon have to deal with many more donor children than originally expected.

One pathway that can lead to the best outcomes for DCP and their donors is one that involves the donor being completely open to allowing their offspring to define and set the boundaries for whatever relationships may result from contact. This sperm donor explains how he puts his offspring in the "driver's seat" when it comes to defining their relationships with him:

After about 5 weeks of conversation, [my donor child] told me that he is going to call me Dad from now on and I am his father because the man who raised him until age 15 was never much of a father and I have been more of a father to him in 5 weeks than that man has been his whole life. Very powerful stuff. I tell them this and will continue to tell them all when we connect: 'I have no expectation of what you will call me and how you will identify me. You will struggle to find what to call me. You will have conflicting feelings regarding this, and it is normal and ok. You may try out whatever you like for as long as you like and you may change it anytime you wish as many times as you like. When you find what works for you, you will feel it.

For donors contacting DCP (or their parents) for the first time, it can be an exciting yet scary experience. Here is some guidance you can share with your client as they go through this process:

- This may be an uncomfortable or overwhelming situation for DCP and their families, even if they have been searching for their donor. Your clients want to get their foot in the door as gently as possible, especially when there is a non-biological parent who might feel threatened.

- Your clients can reassure the DCP or parents that they will allow them to set the boundaries. DCP and their parents should know that your client doesn't want to disrupt their family in any way, that they just want to give them the opportunity to know them and to answer questions. This should be an invitation, not a demand.

- Your clients can let the DCP or parents know that they have thought about them. Many DCP do wonder if the donor has thought about them.

- If your client feels connected enough that it is genuine, let DCP know that they are proud of them. This can be very meaningful for DCP to hear.

- Donors can offer interesting ancestry information and important medical background and updates. They can also tell a little bit about themselves and their family, particularly about their parents and any children they have that are half-siblings to the DCP.

- Donors can share their careers, talents, interests or hobbies, as many DCP will share some of these with them.

- Donors can ask the DCP or their families what type of relationship they'd be open to. A friendship? A more familial relationship? What possibilities are they open to exploring? Donors can tell them why they think this connection could be fulfilling for everyone.

- If a DCP or parent doesn't reply or says "no," it isn't because of who your clients are. It's likely because of their family situation, their lack of emotional bandwidth or a lack of understanding about what connecting might mean for them and their family.

- Donors should understand that in families with non-biological parents, there might be fear associated with connecting to the donor as it might be the first time that the donor is actually acknowledged as a real person and one that has a close genetic connection with their child. DCP with non-biological parents may feel like contact with the donor is a betrayal to their non-bio parent. This is true for DCP with both living and no-longer-living non-biological parents.

- Sometimes, DCP may not respond because of their own physical/mental health issues or fear of not being "good enough."

- Have patience. Sometimes DCP or their parents need some time to work things out internally and with their family members. If your clients get no reply, they can try again in a few weeks or months. If they say no, your clients can let them know they're always available if they change their minds. Donors with biological children under 18 may have to wait until they are over 18 and can then make their own connections. Give them space to hopefully work it out and come around.

The research:

- Many donors feel that it was difficult to judge the appropriate way to develop the relationship.[8]

- A majority limit the number of donor-conceived children that they reach out to.[8]

- Donors who haven't had contact but are interested would prefer that offspring review their profiles, send photos, or communicate by email/text, virtually, and/or meet once (91-97%); and a smaller percent (28-38%) would want to be part of their offspring's daily life.[8]

- Most donors describe their donor-conceived children as a son/daughter or close relative and/or "hard to describe."[8]

- Donors who had contact with their donor-conceived children reported positive experiences and the majority continued to have regular contact.[1,8]

> *Friends come and go, but relatives tend to accumulate.*
> ~ Unknown

I walked out of the weekend meeting with all of my half-siblings and my donor on cloud 9. I had been working in therapy in the weeks leading up to the gathering. What if I didn't like someone? What if they offended me, or we didn't agree on something? This was my "what if" brain working in overdrive ... it was an exciting yet scary weekend to be walking into and I really just wanted the best for everyone involved. My fears melted immediately after meeting everyone. I felt love in the room. We were all curious, maybe a little reserved, but respecting each other, our journeys, and our possible permanent places in each other's lives moving forward. I noticed myself thinking "I love her" about one of my half-sisters not even two hours after knowing her. The thought took me back a bit, but I told myself it's okay to love these people. Everyone that came to the half-siblings gathering that weekend wanted to know their half-siblings, and that leaves a chance of loving your half-siblings. I felt like I could be myself, which is huge because I can be silly and goofy, loud and obnoxious. I felt the same love being given back to me.

None of my fears or anxieties that I had worked out in therapy came to fruition. I couldn't have asked for a better weekend, and I truly feel so blessed that everyone brought their authentic selves to the table for us to learn about and love. -DCP

Connecting is one of the best parts of using donor sperm! It is amazing to see the kids relate, it can be an instant parent support group and it is also amazing to know when medical stuff comes up (glasses, acne, braces). I can not imagine my life without them, or my kids! -Parent

We started connecting with siblings and their families, when our child was 9 months old. We have quite a few hundred in our group...and there are hundreds more we are yet to find, meet and bring into our "family sibling group". The numbers are staggering... However... what I know to be true....is, good or bad (and having 900+ siblings is bad); DC children have a right to know their siblings. Furthermore, these relationships are ideally best fostered as EARLY as possible. Even if it is a Zoom video calling relationship. The connection you see with these kids/siblings is amazing and very moving indeed. -Parent

My biggest point of contention is that I never was able to talk about it with anyone and my conception arrangement has prevented me from ever being able to have a relationship with my biological father, half siblings, grandparents or know the other half of my family history. -DCP

Why would you wait to introduce your child to their brothers and sisters? It is a source of sorrow that my sibling group did not have these opportunities to grow up alongside one another. We missed out on so much. **-DCP**

It's not about feeling unwanted or unloved. For me, it's 2 issues: first, why was I lied to (was told at age 13), and second, why can't I find out who I am. And for me, being loved and wanted is not enough. Because being loved and wanted doesn't answer those burning questions. So help your children find the answers to the questions, and help them to ask the questions, because they may not yet know how to ask. **-DCP**

Like adoptees before them, donor offspring have to decide if they will open themselves up to an honest exploration that may cause them deep sorrow and hurt their existing family relationships, while possibly bringing no tangible benefits, or if they will remain in the protective cocoon of silence or denial, to save themselves the trauma of dealing with the truth. Regardless of the dearth of studies which could effectively quantify serious residual negative issues in the lives of all parties concerned, the potential for such problems cannot be dismissed. **-DCP**

Meeting my donor has been a fascinating experience. Our relationship has changed very little since we first met; I had my questions answered and he was happy to answer them, and what built from there could be likened to a relationship between an Uncle and Nephew who live on opposite ends of the country. We keep in touch and see each other from time to time, but I certainly don't think of him as my "father", nor does he think of me as his "son." We're merely friends who happen to share a very strong genetic connection.

On the other hand, the relationship that I built with my donor grandparents was much stronger; mainly due to the fact that we lived in close geographic proximity. What has evolved over the time that I've known them looks very close to a traditional grandparent/grandchild relationship, albeit one that started much later than most. They truly feel like part of my family and I'm grateful for the opportunity to know them. **-DCP**

One thing is crystal clear for me. That is that the interests and well-being of the children — all of them — are paramount. Regardless of what the legal framework was at the time of my being a sperm donor, I believe that I do have responsibilities to the children born as a result of my sperm donations. At the very least, those children have a right to know what my part of their genetic heritage is. I will be more than happy to get in touch, if and when they do desire. I think about them often and wonder who, where, and how they are, and what is happening in their lives. I think that if one day some of my unknown offspring do make contact with and meet me, it might be — for them primarily and for me too — a wonderful 'jigsaw' experience! All of that said, the prospect of it actually happening is a little daunting, in some ways. What if they do not like me, or I them? What if they feel unhappy with my having contributed to their creation, but then take no responsibility for them — especially if they have had an unhappy life? How will my own family react to and view them? On and on my thinking goes. However, at the base of all of this I am quite clear in my mind, that these wonderful children do have a right to know what they want to know about me — because in them, there is a part of me. **-Sperm Donor**

References

1 Jadva, V., Freeman, T., Kramer, W. & Golombok, S. (2010). Experiences of offspring searching for and contacting their donor siblings and donor. *Reproductive Biomedicine Online*, 20, 523-532. doi:10.1016/j. Rbmo.2010.01.001

2 Hertz, R., Nelson, M. K. & Kramer, W. (2017). Donor sibling networks as a vehicle for expanding kinship: A replication and extension. *Journal of Family Issues*, 38, 248–284, doi: 10.1177/0192513X16631018

3 Frith, L., Sawyer, N. & Kramer, W. (2012). Forming a family with sperm donation: a survey of 244 non-biological parents. *Reproductive Biomedicine Online*, 24, 709-18. doi: 10.1016/j.rbmo.2012.01.013

4 Scheib, J., E. & Ruby, A. (2008). Contact among families who share the same sperm donor. *Fertility & Sterility*, 90, 33-43. doi: 10.1016/j.fertnstert.2007.05.058

5 Beeson, D., Jennings, P.K. & Kramer, W. (2013). A new path to grandparenthood. *Journal of Family Issues*, 34, 1295-1316. doiI:10.1177/0192513X13489299

6 Nelson, M. K., Hertz, R. & Kramer, W. (2013). Making sense of donors and donor siblings: A comparison of the perceptions of donor conceived offspring in lesbian-parent and heterosexual-parent families. In: *Visions of the 21st Century Family: Transforming Structures and Identities Contemporary Perspectives in Family Research*, Volume 7. Emerald Group Publishing Limited.

7 Beeson, D., Kramer, W. & Jennings, P. K. (2011). Offspring searching for their sperm donors: how family type shapes the process. *Human Reproduction*, 26, 2415–2424, doi: https://doi.org/10.1093/humrep/der202

8 Hertz, R., Nelson, M. K. & Kramer, W. (2015). Sperm donors describe the experience of contact with their donor-conceived offspring. Facts, *Views and Vision in Obstetrics and Gynaecology*, 7, 91-100.

9 Scheib, J. E., McCormick, E., Benward, J. & Ruby, A. (2020). Finding people like me: contact among young adults who share an open-identity sperm donor. *Human Reproduction Open*, 2020(4): hoaa057. doi: 10.1093/hropen/hoaa057

Closing

The practice of donor conception is a discipline of medicine where the legacy of secrecy remains in current practice. Given the dramatic increase in the use of these services in recent years, in combination with the Donor Sibling Registry and commercially available tools to easily trace familial DNA, the practice of promised/mandatory anonymity is no longer sustainable. During this long transitional period in the field, we as mental health professionals can assist and empower all donor family members through proper education and counseling, whether this is their primary presenting problem for treatment or it is identified within the context of unrelated issues.

We hope that this guide has been helpful in acquainting you with the most relevant issues so that you can have a better understanding of the complexities and joys that can be found within all donor families. These families, connections, and relationships can be celebrated when all parties can confidently acknowledge the importance of embracing honesty, truth, and each other. Redefining and expanding family can be a joyful experience that you can help to facilitate!

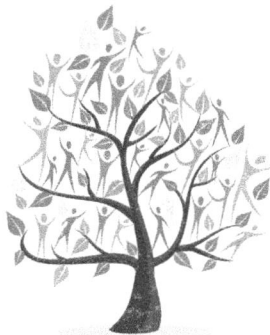

www.ingramcontent.com/pod-product-compliance
Lightning Source LLC
Chambersburg PA
CBHW021434180326
41458CB00001B/262

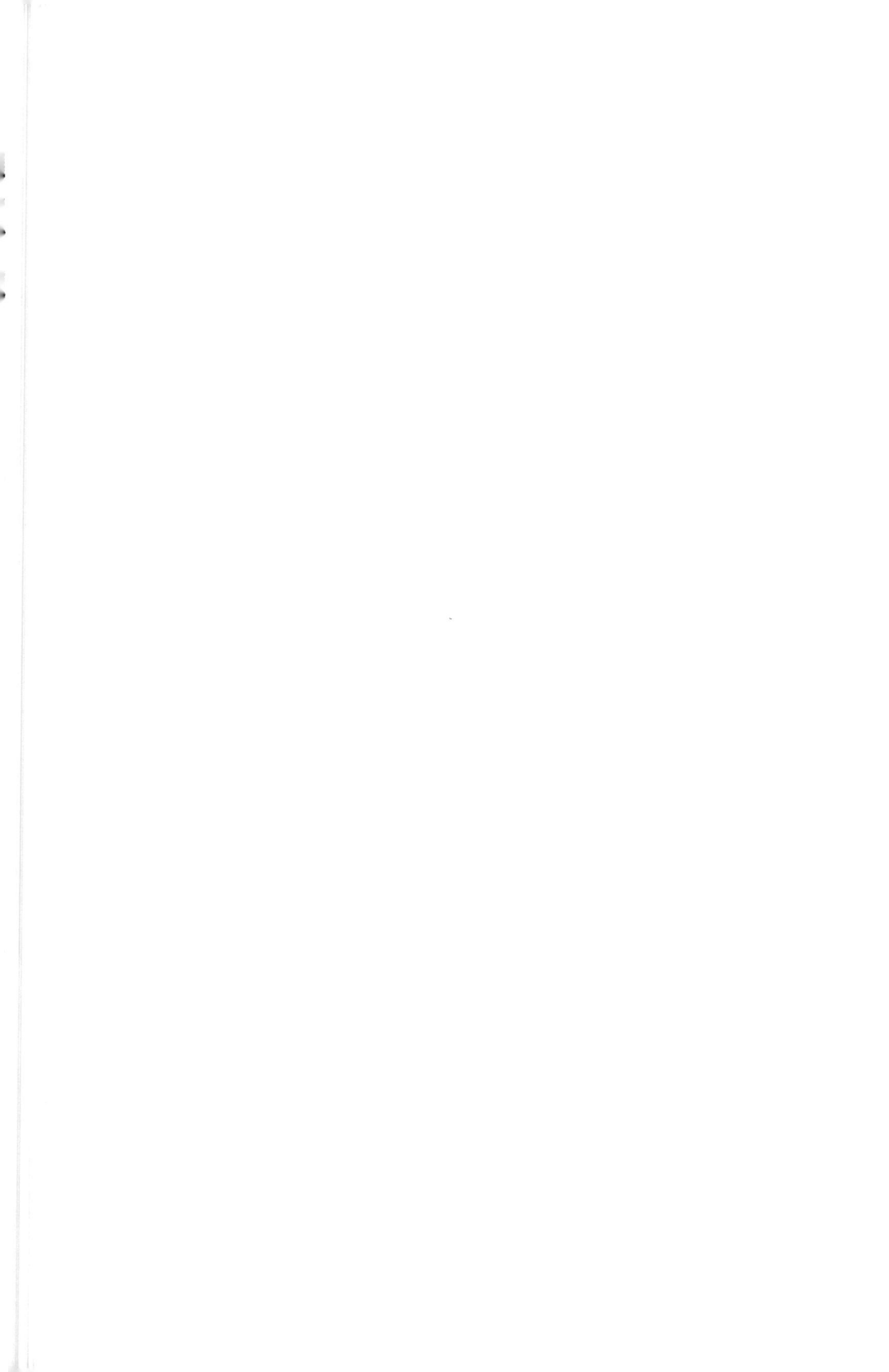